PLANT BASED

COOKBOOK FOR

BEGINNERS

Fuel Your Health, Boost Your Energy, and

Shed Pounds with Nature's Bounty

SAMUEL JONES

TABLE OF CONTENTS

Introduction

Imagine a way of eating that could not only support your health and well-being but also protect the planet we all call home. A diet that provides an abundance of nutrients, fiber, and antioxidants while being gentle on the environment and sustainable for future generations. This is the promise of a plant-based lifestyle, and it's easier than you might think to embrace it.

Whether you're driven by a desire to shed excess weight, boost your energy levels, or reduce your risk of chronic diseases, a plant-based diet has the potential to transform your life. By focusing on whole, minimally processed foods from the earth, you'll be flooding your body with a wide array of vitamins, minerals, and phytochemicals that work in harmony to nourish your cells and optimize your overall health.

But this book isn't just about the "why" of plant-based eating – it's a comprehensive guide to help you seamlessly integrate this way of life into your daily routine. Within these pages, you'll find a wealth of delicious, approachable recipes that prove just how satisfying and flavorful plant-based cuisine can be. From hearty breakfast favorites to nourishing main dishes and decadent desserts, we've got you covered for every meal and occasion.

Gone are the days of bland, unsatisfying meals that leave you feeling deprived. This cookbook is a celebration of the vibrant flavors and textures that nature has to offer, expertly combined to create dishes that are both nutritious and deeply satisfying. With a focus on easy-to-find ingredients and simple techniques, even the most novice cook can confidently whip up these plant-based delights.

Whether you're a longtime vegan, a curious newcomer to this way of eating, or simply looking to incorporate more plant-based meals into your routine, this book is your ultimate guide. Prepare to embark on a journey that will not only delight your taste buds but also leave you feeling energized, radiant, and well on your way to achieving your health and wellness goals.

So, let's dive in and discover the incredible power of plant-based eating – one delicious, nutritious recipe at a time!

Chapter 1

Plant-Based Basics

Why Plant-Based Eating?

Plant-based eating has emerged as a prominent dietary trend in recent years, gaining significant attention from individuals seeking healthier lifestyles, environmental advocates, and animal welfare activists. This shift towards a more plant-centric diet is driven by a multitude of factors, ranging from personal health considerations to ethical and environmental concerns. In the following discussion, we will explore the compelling reasons behind the rise of plant-based eating and its potential benefits.

- **Health Benefits**

One of the primary reasons for embracing a plant-based diet is its potential to promote better overall health. Numerous studies have shown that a diet rich in plant-based foods, such as fruits, vegetables, whole grains, legumes, nuts, and seeds, can help reduce the risk of chronic diseases like heart disease, type 2 diabetes, and certain types of cancer.

Plant-based foods are typically high in fiber, antioxidants, and beneficial plant compounds known as phytochemicals. These nutrients have been linked to various health benefits, including improved digestion, reduced inflammation, better blood sugar control, and a lower risk of obesity.

Additionally, plant-based diets tend to be lower in saturated fats and cholesterol, which can contribute to a healthier cardiovascular system and lower blood pressure levels. By eliminating or reducing the consumption of animal-based products, individuals can potentially reduce their intake of harmful substances like trans fats and hormones often found in processed meats.

- **Environmental Sustainability**

The production of animal-based foods, particularly meat and dairy, has a significant impact on the environment. Animal agriculture is a major contributor to greenhouse gas emissions, deforestation, water pollution, and land degradation.

By adopting a plant-based diet, individuals can significantly reduce their carbon footprint and contribute to a more sustainable food system. Plant-based foods generally require fewer resources, such as water and land, to produce compared to animal-based products.

Furthermore, the livestock industry is a major driver of deforestation, as vast areas of forests are cleared to make way for grazing lands and the cultivation of animal feed crops. By reducing the demand for animal-based products, we can help protect vital ecosystems and biodiversity.

- **Animal Welfare**

For many individuals, the ethical treatment of animals is a driving force behind their decision to adopt a plant-based diet. Factory farming practices, which prioritize efficiency and cost-effectiveness over animal welfare, often subject animals to cramped living conditions, painful procedures, and inhumane treatment.

By eliminating or reducing the consumption of animal-based products, individuals can take a stance against these practices and reduce the demand for industrialized animal agriculture. Plant-based diets offer a compassionate alternative that minimizes the suffering of sentient beings.

- **Food Security and Accessibility**

As the global population continues to grow, the demand for food sources that are sustainable, efficient, and accessible becomes increasingly important. Plant-based foods have the potential to address food security and accessibility challenges more effectively than animal-based products.

Plant-based foods are generally more resource-efficient and require less land, water, and energy to produce compared to animal-based foods. This makes plant-based diets a more viable option for feeding a growing global population while minimizing the strain on natural resources.

Additionally, many plant-based foods are locally grown and culturally diverse, ensuring their availability and accessibility to a wider range of communities worldwide.

- **Personal Ethics and Values**

For some individuals, the decision to adopt a plant-based diet is rooted in personal ethics and values. This dietary choice may align with religious or spiritual beliefs, cultural traditions, or a personal commitment to living a more mindful and compassionate lifestyle.

Plant-based diets can be an expression of respect for life, a desire to minimize harm to living beings, and a rejection of exploitative practices associated with industrialized animal agriculture.

- **Culinary Exploration and Variety**

Contrary to the misconception that plant-based diets are restrictive, many individuals find joy and excitement in exploring the vast array of plant-based cuisines from around the world. Plant-based eating offers an opportunity to discover new flavors, textures, and culinary techniques that celebrate the diversity and versatility of plant-based ingredients.

From hearty lentil stews to vibrant vegetable curries, from flavorful veggie burgers to decadent plant-based desserts, the plant-based culinary world is vast and constantly evolving. This exploration can not only nourish the body but also ignite a passion for food and nutrition.

The reasons behind the rise of plant-based eating are multifaceted, encompassing health considerations, environmental sustainability, animal welfare concerns, food security, personal ethics, and culinary exploration. As more individuals recognize the potential benefits of a plant-centric diet, this dietary trend is likely to continue gaining momentum, shaping the way we think about food production, consumption, and our relationship with the natural world.

Benefits of a Plant-Based Diet

Embracing a plant-based diet can lead to numerous benefits that extend far beyond personal health. This dietary approach, which emphasizes the consumption of whole, minimally processed plant foods, has gained significant traction in recent years due to its potential positive impact on various aspects of our lives and the world around us. In this comprehensive discussion, we will explore the multifaceted advantages of adopting a plant-based diet.

- **Improved Overall Health**

One of the most compelling benefits of a plant-based diet is its potential to enhance overall health and well-being. Numerous studies have consistently demonstrated that individuals following a plant-based diet tend to have a lower risk of developing chronic diseases such as heart disease, type 2 diabetes, certain types of cancer, and obesity.

Plant-based foods are naturally rich in fiber, antioxidants, phytochemicals, and other beneficial nutrients that can help reduce inflammation, improve digestion, and support a healthy immune system. By eliminating or minimizing the consumption of animal-based products, which are often high in saturated fats and cholesterol, individuals can potentially lower their risk of developing cardiovascular issues and improve their blood lipid profiles.

Furthermore, plant-based diets have been associated with better weight management and a reduced risk of obesity. This can be attributed to the fact that plant-based foods are typically lower in calories and higher in fiber, promoting a feeling of fullness and satiety, which can aid in portion control and prevent overeating.

- **Environmental Sustainability**

The production of animal-based foods, particularly meat and dairy, has a significant environmental impact. Animal agriculture is a major contributor to greenhouse gas emissions, deforestation, water pollution, and land degradation. By adopting a plant-based diet, individuals can significantly reduce their carbon footprint and contribute to a more sustainable food system.

Plant-based foods generally require fewer resources, such as water and land, to produce compared to animal-based products. Additionally, the livestock industry is a major driver of deforestation, as vast areas of forests are cleared to make way for grazing lands and the cultivation of animal feed crops. By reducing the demand for animal-based products, we can help protect vital ecosystems and biodiversity.

Moreover, the transportation and distribution of plant-based foods often have a lower environmental impact compared to the transportation of livestock and their associated products, further reducing the carbon footprint of a plant-based diet.

- **Animal Welfare Considerations**

For many individuals, the ethical treatment of animals is a driving force behind their decision to adopt a plant-based diet. Factory farming practices, which prioritize efficiency and cost-effectiveness over animal welfare, often subject animals to cramped living conditions, painful procedures, and inhumane treatment.

By eliminating or reducing the consumption of animal-based products, individuals can take a stance against these practices and reduce the demand for industrialized animal agriculture. Plant-based diets offer a compassionate alternative that minimizes the suffering of sentient beings and aligns with the principles of compassion and respect for all life forms.

- **Food Security and Accessibility**

As the global population continues to grow, the demand for food sources that are sustainable, efficient, and accessible becomes increasingly important. Plant-based foods have the potential to address food security and accessibility challenges more effectively than animal-based products.

Plant-based foods are generally more resource-efficient and require less land, water, and energy to produce compared to animal-based foods. This makes plant-based diets a more viable option for feeding a growing global population while minimizing the strain on natural resources.

Additionally, many plant-based foods are locally grown and culturally diverse, ensuring their availability and accessibility to a wider range of communities worldwide. This can contribute to improved food security and reduce dependence on imported or industrialized food sources.

- **Personal Ethics and Values**

For some individuals, the decision to adopt a plant-based diet is rooted in personal ethics and values. This dietary choice may align with religious or spiritual beliefs, cultural traditions, or a personal commitment to living a more mindful and compassionate lifestyle.

Plant-based diets can be an expression of respect for life, a desire to minimize harm to living beings, and a rejection of exploitative practices associated with industrialized animal agriculture. By adopting a plant-based diet, individuals can live in alignment with their ethical principles and contribute to a more compassionate world.

- **Culinary Exploration and Variety**

Contrary to the misconception that plant-based diets are restrictive, many individuals find joy and excitement in exploring the vast array of plant-based cuisines from around the world. Plant-based eating offers an opportunity to discover new flavors, textures, and culinary techniques that celebrate the diversity and versatility of plant-based ingredients.

From hearty lentil stews to vibrant vegetable curries, from flavorful veggie burgers to decadent plant-based desserts, the plant-based culinary world is vast and constantly evolving. This exploration can not only nourish the body but also ignite a passion for food and nutrition, encouraging individuals to embrace a more diverse and exciting approach to meal preparation.

- **Potential Cost Savings**

While the perception may exist that a plant-based diet is more expensive, in reality, it can often be a more cost-effective way of eating. Plant-based staples such as grains, legumes, and many fruits and vegetables tend to be more affordable than animal-based products, especially when purchased in bulk or from local sources.

Additionally, by reducing or eliminating the consumption of processed and packaged foods, which are often more expensive, individuals can potentially save money while also promoting better health. The long-term benefits of a plant-based diet, such as reduced healthcare costs associated with chronic diseases, can also contribute to overall cost savings.

The benefits of a plant-based diet are multifaceted and far-reaching. From promoting better overall health and reducing the risk of chronic diseases to contributing to environmental sustainability and addressing ethical considerations, adopting a plant-based approach to eating can have a profound impact on both personal well-being and the world around us. As awareness of these benefits continues to grow, more individuals may be inspired to embrace a plant-based lifestyle, creating a positive ripple effect that extends beyond personal choices and into the realms of sustainability, compassion, and global well-being.

Common Myths and Misconceptions

The plant-based diet, while gaining increasing popularity and recognition for its numerous benefits, is still surrounded by several myths and misconceptions. These misconceptions often stem from a lack of understanding, outdated information, or deeply ingrained societal norms. In this discussion, we will address and debunk some of the most common myths and misconceptions associated with plant-based eating.

Myth: Plant-based diets are deficient in essential nutrients. One of the most prevalent misconceptions about plant-based diets is the notion that they are inherently deficient in essential nutrients, particularly protein, iron, calcium, and vitamin B12. However, this belief is unfounded and fails to recognize the abundance and variety of nutrient-rich plant-based foods available.

Contrary to popular belief, plant-based diets can provide all the necessary nutrients for optimal health when carefully planned and balanced. Proteins can be obtained from a variety of sources, including legumes, grains, nuts, seeds, and even some vegetables. Iron is present in foods like lentils, spinach, cashews, and fortified plant-based milks. Calcium can be found in leafy greens, tofu, tempeh, and fortified plant-based products. Additionally, vitamin B12, which is primarily produced by bacteria, can be obtained through fortified foods or supplements.

By incorporating a diverse range of plant-based foods and ensuring proper meal planning, individuals can easily meet their nutritional needs without relying on animal-based products.

Myth: Plant-based diets lack flavor and variety. Another common misconception is that plant-based diets are bland, boring, and lacking in variety. This belief often stems from a limited understanding of the vast culinary possibilities that plant-based eating offers.

In reality, the plant-based culinary world is rich, diverse, and full of exciting flavors and textures. From the bold spices of Indian curries to the umami-packed flavors of Asian cuisine, from the vibrant colors and aromas of Mediterranean dishes to the comforting and hearty stews of Latin American cuisine, plant-based cooking embraces a wide range of cultural traditions and culinary techniques.

With the abundance of fruits, vegetables, grains, legumes, nuts, seeds, and plant-based proteins available, the possibilities for creating flavorful and satisfying meals are endless. Additionally, the rise of plant-based alternatives and innovative products has further expanded the culinary horizons, offering plant-based versions of traditional favorites like burgers, sausages, and even cheeses.

Myth: Plant-based diets are expensive and inaccessible. There is a perception that following a plant-based diet is inherently more expensive and inaccessible, particularly for those with limited financial resources. However, this myth fails to consider the true affordability and accessibility of plant-based foods.

Many plant-based staples, such as grains, legumes, and many fruits and vegetables, are among the most budget-friendly options available. When purchased in bulk or from local sources, these ingredients can be incredibly cost-effective. Additionally, by reducing reliance on processed and packaged foods, individuals can save money while promoting better health.

Furthermore, plant-based diets are not exclusive to specific cultures or socioeconomic backgrounds. Many traditional cuisines around the world are heavily plant-based, relying on locally sourced and culturally significant ingredients. This makes plant-based eating accessible to diverse communities and helps to preserve cultural traditions and food heritage.

Myth: Plant-based diets are restrictive and difficult to maintain. Some individuals perceive plant-based diets as overly restrictive and challenging to maintain, particularly in social settings or when dining out. However, this misconception fails to acknowledge the flexibility and adaptability of plant-based eating.

With the growing popularity of plant-based lifestyles, many restaurants and food establishments now offer a variety of plant-based options, making it easier than ever to find satisfying and delicious meals while dining out. Additionally, with the rise of plant-based alternatives and meat substitutes, individuals can still enjoy familiar flavors and textures without relying on animal-based products.

Furthermore, plant-based diets can be tailored to individual preferences and dietary needs, allowing for flexibility and personal customization. From strict veganism to more flexible plant-based approaches that include occasional animal-based products, individuals can find a dietary pattern that aligns with their values, goals, and lifestyles.

Myth: Plant-based diets are unsuitable for athletes and active individuals. There is a persistent myth that plant-based diets are inadequate for meeting the nutritional demands of athletes and highly active individuals. This belief stems from the misconception that plant-based foods cannot provide sufficient protein, energy, and other essential nutrients for optimal performance and recovery.

However, numerous studies and the experiences of successful plant-based athletes have challenged this notion. When properly planned and balanced, plant-based diets can provide all the necessary macronutrients (proteins, carbohydrates, and healthy fats) and micronutrients required for athletic performance, muscle recovery, and overall physical well-being.

Plant-based protein sources, such as soy, legumes, grains, and plant-based protein powders, can adequately support muscle growth and repair. Additionally, carbohydrate-rich plant-based foods like whole grains, fruits, and vegetables can provide the energy needed for endurance and high-intensity activities.

Myth: Plant-based diets are a temporary fad or trend. Some individuals perceive plant-based diets as a passing fad or trend, dismissing their long-term viability and relevance. However, this belief fails to recognize the deep-rooted and multifaceted reasons behind the growing popularity of plant-based eating.

Plant-based diets are not just a fleeting trend but a dietary approach rooted in ethical, environmental, and health considerations. As awareness of the impact of our food choices on personal well-being, animal welfare, and environmental sustainability grows, more individuals are embracing plant-based eating as a conscious and lasting lifestyle choice.

Furthermore, the scientific evidence supporting the health benefits of plant-based diets continues to accumulate, solidifying their place as a legitimate and sustainable dietary pattern. With the ongoing advancements in plant-based food technology and the increasing availability of plant-based options, plant-based eating is poised to become a mainstream and enduring dietary choice.

The myths and misconceptions surrounding plant-based diets often stem from a lack of understanding, outdated information, or ingrained societal norms. By addressing and debunking these misconceptions, we can promote a more informed and balanced dialogue around plant-based eating.

Recognizing the abundance, variety, and nutritional adequacy of plant-based foods, as well as the ethical, environmental, and health implications of our dietary choices, can help individuals make more informed decisions and embrace plant-based eating as a viable and sustainable lifestyle.

Essential Ingredients for a Plant-Based Kitchen

Transitioning to a plant-based diet requires a well-stocked kitchen with a variety of wholesome, nutrient-dense ingredients. While the options may seem overwhelming at first, having a solid foundation of essential plant-based ingredients can make meal planning and preparation a breeze. In this discussion, we will explore the key components that should be staples in any plant-based kitchen, providing a comprehensive guide to building a diverse and flavorful plant-based pantry.

- **Whole Grains**

Whole grains are an indispensable part of a plant-based diet, providing a rich source of complex carbohydrates, fiber, vitamins, and minerals. Some essential whole grains to stock up on include:

❖ Brown rice: A versatile and nutrient-dense option that can be used in countless dishes, from stir-fries to pilafs.

❖ Quinoa: A gluten-free pseudograin that's high in protein and fiber, making it a great addition to salads, bowls, and stuffed vegetables.

❖ Oats: Both rolled and steel-cut oats are excellent for breakfast porridges, granolas, and baked goods.

❖ Whole wheat pasta: A nutritious alternative to traditional refined pasta, offering a satisfying chew and a nutty flavor.

❖ Farro, barley, and bulgur: These ancient grains add texture and depth to soups, salads, and pilafs.

- **Legumes**

Legumes, such as beans, lentils, and peas, are essential in a plant-based kitchen as they provide a rich source of plant-based protein, fiber, and various essential nutrients. Some must-have legumes include:

- ❖ Chickpeas: Versatile and packed with protein, chickpeas can be used in everything from hummus to curries and salads.

- ❖ Lentils: Available in a variety of colors, lentils are a nutritious and convenient source of protein that can be easily incorporated into soups, stews, and patties.

- ❖ Black beans, kidney beans, and pinto beans: These hearty beans can be used in chili, burritos, and rice dishes.

- ❖ Split peas: Perfect for making thick, creamy soups and dips.

- **Nuts and Seeds**

  Nuts and seeds are nutrient powerhouses that provide healthy fats, proteins, and an array of vitamins and minerals. Some essential options to have on hand include:

- ❖ Almonds, cashews, and walnuts: Excellent for snacking, baking, and adding crunch to salads and stir-fries.

- ❖ Chia seeds and flaxseeds: These tiny seeds are rich in omega-3 fatty acids and fiber, making them ideal for adding to smoothies, oatmeal, and baked goods.

- ❖ Pumpkin seeds and sunflower seeds: Packed with protein and minerals, these seeds can be used as a topping for salads, soups, and even plant-based yogurt parfaits.

- **Fresh Produce**

A plant-based diet revolves around the vibrant and nutrient-rich world of fresh fruits and vegetables. Stocking up on a variety of seasonal produce is key to creating flavorful and nutritious meals. Some essential items to have on hand include:

- ❖ Leafy greens: Spinach, kale, Swiss chard, and arugula are versatile and nutrient-dense options for salads, smoothies, and sautés.

- ❖ Cruciferous vegetables: Broccoli, cauliflower, Brussels sprouts, and cabbage are packed with fiber, vitamins, and antioxidants.

❖ Vegetables for roasting: Sweet potatoes, carrots, beets, and bell peppers are perfect for roasting and adding to grain bowls or salads.

❖ Fresh herbs: Cilantro, parsley, basil, and rosemary can elevate the flavor of any plant-based dish.

❖ Fruits: Bananas, apples, oranges, berries, and avocados offer a natural sweetness and plenty of nutrients.

• **Plant-Based Proteins**

While legumes and grains provide a good source of plant-based protein, having additional options can add variety and convenience to your plant-based meals.

Some essential plant-based protein sources to consider include:

❖ Tofu and tempeh: These soy-based products are incredibly versatile and can be used in stir-fries, curries, and even plant-based "meat" dishes.

❖ Seitan: Made from wheat gluten, seitan has a meat-like texture and can be seasoned and prepared in various ways.

❖ Plant-based meat alternatives: With the rise of plant-based companies, the market now offers a wide range of meatless burgers, sausages, and other meat substitutes.

- **Condiments and Seasonings**

Flavorful condiments and seasonings are essential for adding depth and complexity to plant-based dishes. Some must-have items include:

* Spices: Cumin, chili powder, paprika, turmeric, and curry powder can instantly elevate the flavor of any dish.

* Herbs: Dried basil, oregano, thyme, and rosemary are versatile and can be used in a variety of cuisines.

* Vinegars: Balsamic, apple cider, and red wine vinegars can add tanginess and depth to dressings, marinades, and sauces.

- ❖ Soy sauce, tamari, or coconut aminos: These umami-rich condiments are perfect for seasoning stir-fries, marinades, and sauces.

- ❖ Nut and seed butter: Almond, peanut, and tahini (sesame seed paste) can be used in dressings, sauces, and baked goods.

Plant-Based Milks and Dairy

Alternatives: For those looking to eliminate or reduce their consumption of dairy products, plant-based milks and dairy alternatives are essential. Some options to consider include:

- ❖ Plant-based milks: Almond, soy, oat, and coconut milks can be used for drinking, cooking, and baking.

❖ Plant-based yogurt: Made from various plant sources like soy, coconut, or almonds, these yogurts can be enjoyed as a snack or used in dips and dressings.

❖ Plant-based cheese: From nut-based spreads to cashew-based cheeses, these alternatives can satisfy cravings for cheese while adhering to a plant-based diet.

- **Whole Food Starches**

  While often overlooked, whole food starches can be an excellent source of energy, fiber, and essential nutrients in a plant-based diet. Some options to have on hand include:

❖ Potatoes: Sweet potatoes, Yukon Gold, and Russet potatoes can be baked, roasted, or mashed for a satisfying and nutrient-dense side dish.

❖ Corn: Fresh corn on the cob or frozen corn kernels can be added to salads, soups, and chili.

❖ Winter squash: Acorn, butternut, and pumpkin are rich in vitamins and can be roasted, pureed, or added to soups and stews.

By stocking your plant-based kitchen with these essential ingredients, you'll have a solid foundation for creating delicious, nutritious, and satisfying meals. Remember, the key to a successful plant-based diet is variety, balance, and creativity. Don't be afraid to experiment with new ingredients, flavors, and cuisines, as the world of plant-based eating is vast and ever-evolving.

Kitchen Tools and Equipment

Adopting a plant-based diet often requires a shift in kitchen tools and equipment to accommodate the preparation and cooking methods of plant-based ingredients. While some tools may already be present in your kitchen, others may need to be acquired or upgraded to streamline the process of creating delicious and nutritious plant-based meals. In this part, we will explore the essential kitchen tools and equipment that can help make your plant-based culinary journey more efficient and enjoyable.

- **High-quality pots and pans**

  Investing in a good set of pots and pans is crucial for any kitchen, but it becomes even more important when following a plant-based diet. Opt for durable, non-toxic cookware that can withstand high heat and distribute it evenly. Stainless steel, cast iron, and ceramic-coated pots and pans are excellent choices for sautéing vegetables, simmering soups and stews, and cooking grains and legumes.

- **Sharp knives**

  A high-quality chef's knife and a paring knife are essential tools for any plant-based kitchen. With the abundance of fresh produce and vegetables involved in plant-based cooking, having sharp knives will make chopping, slicing, and dicing a breeze. Invest in knives with comfortable handles and sharp, durable blades to ensure precision and safety during food preparation.

- **Food processor and blender**

A food processor and a high-powered blender are invaluable tools for plant-based cooking. A food processor can be used for tasks such as grinding nuts and seeds, making nut butters, chopping vegetables, and even preparing plant-based doughs and batters. A blender, on the other hand, is perfect for creating smooth and creamy textures, like

plant-based milks, soups, sauces, and
smoothies.

- **Spiralizer or vegetable slicer**

A spiralizer or vegetable slicer is a handy tool
that can transform vegetables into noodle-
like shapes, adding variety and creativity to
your plant-based meals. These tools can turn
vegetables like zucchini, sweet potatoes, and
beets into "noodles" that can be used as a
substitute for traditional pasta or as a base for
salads and stir-fries.

- **Oven-safe baking dishes**

Plant-based baking often involves the use of
alternative ingredients like nuts, seeds, and
plant-based milks. Having a selection of

oven-safe baking dishes, such as loaf pans, pie plates, and casserole dishes, will allow you to explore a wide range of plant-based baked goods, from breads and cakes to savory dishes like roasted vegetables and baked casseroles.

- **Baking sheets and silicone mats**
Baking sheets and silicone mats are essential for roasting vegetables, baking plant-based patties or burgers, and preparing crispy tofu or tempeh. Look for rimmed baking sheets that can accommodate a large quantity of ingredients, and invest in silicone mats or parchment paper to prevent sticking and ensure easy cleanup.

- **Graters and zesters**

  Graters and zesters are versatile tools that can add flavor and texture to your plant-based dishes. Use a box grater to shred vegetables like carrots or beets for salads or to create plant-based "cheese" from nuts or seeds. A zester can help you extract the aromatic oils from citrus fruits, adding a burst of fresh flavor to dressings, sauces, and marinades.

- **Spice grinder or mortar and pestle**

  A spice grinder or mortar and pestle can be invaluable for grinding whole spices and creating custom spice blends. Freshly ground spices can elevate the flavor of your plant-based dishes and add depth and complexity to sauces, marinades, and rubs.

- **Steamer basket or steamer pot**

  Steaming is a healthy and efficient way to cook vegetables while preserving their nutrients and flavor. A steamer basket or steamer pot can be used to steam vegetables, dumplings, or even plant-based proteins like tofu or tempeh, resulting in tender and flavorful dishes.

- **High-quality storage containers**

  Proper storage is essential for keeping plant-based ingredients fresh and reducing food waste. Invest in airtight containers of various sizes to store dry goods like grains, nuts, and seeds, as well as reusable containers for storing leftovers or prepped ingredients in the refrigerator or freezer.

- **Instant Pot or pressure cooker**

An Instant Pot or pressure cooker can be a game-changer for plant-based cooking, especially when it comes to preparing beans, lentils, and whole grains. These appliances drastically reduce cooking times, making it easier to incorporate these nutrient-dense ingredients into your daily meals.

- **High-speed immersion blender**

A high-speed immersion blender is a versatile tool that can be used to blend soups, sauces, and dips directly in the pot or bowl, eliminating the need for transferring hot liquids to a traditional blender. This tool is particularly useful for creating smooth and creamy plant-based soups and purees.

- **Dehydrator**

  While not an essential tool, a dehydrator can be a valuable addition to a plant-based kitchen. It allows you to create your own plant-based snacks, like dehydrated fruit leathers, vegetable chips, and even plant-based "jerky" from ingredients like mushrooms or eggplant.

- **Waffle iron or griddle**

  For those who enjoy plant-based breakfast options, a waffle iron or griddle can open up a world of possibilities. From fluffy vegan waffles to savory plant-based pancakes, these tools can help you create satisfying and nutritious morning meals.

- **Mason jars and reusable bottles**

Mason jars and reusable bottles can serve multiple purposes in a plant-based kitchen. They can be used for storing homemade plant-based milks, dressings, and sauces, as well as for transporting smoothies or juices on-the-go. Investing in a variety of sizes can make meal preparation and storage more convenient and eco-friendly.

While this list covers many essential tools and equipment, it's important to remember that a plant-based kitchen is flexible and can be adapted to your individual needs and preferences. Start with the basics and gradually build your collection as your culinary skills and interests evolve. With the right tools and equipment, you can unlock a world of plant-based culinary possibilities, making the transition to a plant-based diet more enjoyable and sustainable.

Tips for Meal Planning and Prep

Adopting a plant-based diet can be a transformative journey, offering numerous benefits for your health, the environment, and ethical considerations. However, successful meal planning and preparation are crucial to ensuring a smooth transition and long-term adherence to this lifestyle. Here, we will explore practical tips and strategies for meal planning and prep that will streamline your plant-based journey and make it more enjoyable and sustainable.

- **Start with a well-stocked pantry and fridge**

Having a well-stocked pantry and fridge is the foundation for efficient meal planning and prep. Make sure to have a variety of plant-based staples on hand, such as whole grains, legumes, nuts, seeds, and a diverse selection of fresh fruits and vegetables. This will not only provide you with a range of options but also inspire creativity in your meal planning.

- **Batch cooking and meal prepping**

  One of the keys to success in a plant-based lifestyle is meal prepping. Set aside dedicated time each week to batch cook grains, legumes, and roasted vegetables. These can then be easily incorporated into meals throughout the week, saving you time and effort during busy weeknights. Additionally, consider prepping plant-based snacks, such as energy balls, hummus, or veggie sticks, to have on hand for when hunger strikes.

- **Meal planning and scheduling**

Create a weekly meal plan that incorporates a variety of plant-based dishes. This will not only help you stay organized and avoid last-minute scrambles but also ensure that you're getting a balanced intake of nutrients. Consider planning meals around specific ingredients or themes, such as "Meatless Monday," "Taco Tuesday," or "Buddha Bowl Wednesday," to keep things interesting and exciting.

- **Utilize leftovers creatively**

Plant-based cooking often results in larger portions, which can be a blessing in disguise. Embrace leftovers and find creative ways to repurpose them into new dishes. For example, leftover roasted vegetables can be transformed into a stir-fry, salad, or even a savory breakfast hash. Leftover grains can be used to create grain bowls or added to soups and stews.

- **Invest in meal prep containers**

  Having a set of high-quality, airtight meal prep containers can make a world of difference in your plant-based meal planning. These containers not only help you portion out meals and snacks but also ensure that your food stays fresh and maintains its texture and flavor. Look for containers that are microwave-safe, leak-proof, and stackable for easy storage.

- **Embrace plant-based convenience foods**

  While cooking from scratch is often preferred, there's no need to shy away from plant-based convenience foods. Having a selection of frozen or pre-made plant-based options, such as veggie burgers, faux meats, or ready-to-eat meals, can be a lifesaver on busy days or when you're short on time. These products can be incorporated into your meal planning and serve as a quick and easy backup.

- **Experiment with new recipes and cuisines**

  One of the joys of a plant-based diet is the opportunity to explore a wide range of cuisines and flavors. Challenge yourself to try new recipes and ingredients each week, whether it's a Middle Eastern lentil dish, a Thai coconut curry, or a Mexican-inspired veggie bowl. This will not only add variety to your meals but also expose you to different cultural cuisines and cooking techniques.

- **Invest in time-saving kitchen tools**

  Certain kitchen tools and appliances can significantly streamline your meal prep process. Consider investing in a high-quality blender for making smoothies and plant-based milks, a food processor for chopping vegetables and making dips, or an Instant Pot or pressure cooker for quickly cooking grains and legumes. These tools can save you valuable time and effort in the kitchen.

- **Plan for snacks and on-the-go options**

A plant-based lifestyle doesn't have to be confined to your home. Plan for snacks and on-the-go options to ensure you're never caught off guard when hunger strikes. Pack portable snacks like fresh fruit, trail mixes, energy bars, or veggie wraps for when you're on the move. Additionally, research plant-based options at nearby restaurants or cafes for those times when you're dining out.

- **Involve family and friends**

Meal planning and prep can be more enjoyable and sustainable when you involve your loved ones. Get your family or friends involved in the process by sharing recipe ideas, shopping together, or hosting plant-based potlucks or cooking sessions. This not only fosters a sense of community but also provides support and encouragement along your plant-based journey.

- **Utilize meal planning apps and resources**
  In today's digital age, there are numerous meal planning apps and online resources available to help streamline your plant-based journey. These tools can provide recipe ideas, generate grocery lists, and even suggest meal plans based on your dietary preferences and goals. Explore options like Planty, Forks

Over Knives, or Plant-Based Meal Planner to find the right fit for your needs.

- **Stay organized and flexible**

  While meal planning and prep can bring structure and organization to your plant-based lifestyle, it's essential to remain flexible. Life can be unpredictable, and your plans may need to adjust accordingly. Don't be too rigid in your approach, and allow room for spontaneity and adjustments when necessary. The key is to have a solid foundation and a backup plan for those unexpected situations.

- **Focus on nutrient-dense foods**

When planning your plant-based meals, prioritize nutrient-dense foods that offer a wide range of vitamins, minerals, fiber, and healthy fats. Incorporate a variety of colorful fruits and vegetables, whole grains, legumes, nuts, and seeds into your meals to ensure you're meeting your nutritional needs.

- **Plan for special occasions and holidays**

Special occasions and holidays can present unique challenges when it comes to sticking to a plant-based diet. Plan ahead by researching plant-based recipes or dishes that can be incorporated into these celebrations. Additionally, communicate your dietary preferences with hosts or family members to ensure there are suitable options available.

- **Be patient and celebrate small wins**

  Transitioning to a plant-based lifestyle can be a journey, and it's essential to be patient with yourself and celebrate small wins along the way. Recognize and acknowledge the positive changes you've made, whether it's trying a new plant-based recipe or successfully meal prepping for the week. These small victories will help keep you motivated and inspired on your plant-based path.

By implementing these tips and strategies, you'll be well-equipped to navigate the world of plant-based meal planning and prep with confidence and ease. Remember, the key to success lies in being organized, creative, and flexible. Embrace the process, experiment with new flavors and cuisines, and enjoy the nourishing and delicious plant-based meals you create.

Chapter 2

Breakfast Delights

Green Smoothie Bowl

Description: A refreshing and nutritious blend of green fruits and vegetables topped with your favorite toppings.

Preparation time: 10 minutes

Cooking time: 0 minutes

Number of servings: 2

Ingredients:

- 2 cups fresh spinach leaves

- 1 ripe banana, peeled and sliced

- 1 cup frozen mango chunks

- 1/2 avocado, peeled and pitted

- 1/2 cup plain Greek yogurt

- 1 tablespoon honey or maple syrup (optional)

- 1/2 cup almond milk or any milk of your choice

Toppings (optional):

- Sliced fresh fruits (e.g., banana, kiwi, berries)

- Granola

- Chia seeds

- Coconut flakes

- Nut butter

How to make:

1. In a blender, combine spinach, banana, mango, avocado, Greek yogurt, honey or maple syrup (if using), and almond milk.

2. Blend until smooth and creamy, adding more milk if needed to reach your desired consistency.

3. Pour the smoothie into bowls and top with your favorite toppings.

4. Serve immediately and enjoy!

   Nutritional info: (per serving)

- Calories: 250

- Protein: 10g

- Fat: 7g

- Carbohydrates: 45g

- Fiber: 8g

Tropical Mango Smoothie

Description: A vibrant and tropical blend of ripe mangoes and coconut for a taste of paradise.

Preparation time: 5 minutes

Cooking time: 0 minutes

Number of servings: 2

Ingredients:

- 2 cups frozen mango chunks

- 1 ripe banana, peeled

- 1/2 cup coconut milk

- 1/2 cup plain Greek yogurt

- 1 tablespoon honey or maple syrup (optional)

- Juice of 1 lime

How to make:

1. In a blender, combine frozen mango chunks, banana, coconut milk, Greek yogurt, honey or maple syrup (if using), and lime juice.

2. Blend until smooth and creamy.

3. Pour into glasses and serve immediately.

Nutritional info: (per serving)

- Calories: 220

- Protein: 6g

- Fat: 6g

- Carbohydrates: 40g

- Fiber: 5g

Blueberry Almond Butter Smoothie

Description: A creamy and antioxidant-rich smoothie featuring the delightful flavor combination of blueberries and almond butter.

Preparation time: 5 minutes

Cooking time: 0 minutes

Number of servings: 2

Ingredients:

- 2 cups frozen blueberries

- 1 ripe banana, peeled

- 2 tablespoons almond butter

- 1 cup almond milk or any milk of your choice

- 1/2 cup plain Greek yogurt

- 1 tablespoon honey or maple syrup (optional)

How to make:

1. In a blender, combine frozen blueberries, banana, almond butter, almond milk, Greek yogurt, and honey or maple syrup (if using).

2. Blend until smooth and creamy.

3. Pour into glasses and serve immediately.

Nutritional info: (per serving)

- Calories: 280

- Protein: 9g

- Fat: 10g

- Carbohydrates: 45g

- Fiber: 8g

Peanut Butter Banana Smoothie Bowl

Description: A satisfying and protein-packed smoothie bowl featuring the classic combination of peanut butter and banana.

Preparation time: 10 minutes

Cooking time: 0 minutes

Number of servings: 2

Ingredients:

- 2 ripe bananas, peeled and sliced

- 2 tablespoons peanut butter

- 1 cup plain Greek yogurt

- 1/2 cup almond milk or any milk of your choice

- 1 tablespoon honey or maple syrup (optional)

- Toppings (optional):

- Sliced bananas

- Granola

- Chia seeds

- Peanut butter drizzle

How to make:

1. In a blender, combine sliced bananas, peanut butter, Greek yogurt, almond milk, and honey or maple syrup (if using).

2. Blend until smooth and creamy.

3. Pour the smoothie into bowls and add your favorite toppings.

4. Serve immediately and enjoy!

Nutritional info: (per serving)

- Calories: 320

- Protein: 15g

- Fat: 12g

- Carbohydrates: 45g

- Fiber: 6g

Strawberry Coconut Smoothie

Description: A delightful blend of sweet strawberries and creamy coconut milk for a refreshing treat.

Preparation time: 5 minutes

Cooking time: 0 minutes

Number of servings: 2

Ingredients:

- 2 cups frozen strawberries

- 1 ripe banana, peeled

- 1/2 cup coconut milk

- 1/2 cup plain Greek yogurt

- 1 tablespoon honey or maple syrup (optional)

How to make:

1. In a blender, combine frozen strawberries, banana, coconut milk, Greek yogurt, and honey or maple syrup (if using).

2. Blend until smooth and creamy.

3. Pour into glasses and serve immediately.

Nutritional info: (per serving)

- Calories: 200

- Protein: 6g

- Fat: 5g

- Carbohydrates: 35g

- Fiber: 6g

Overnight Oats with Mixed Berries

Description: A simple and nutritious breakfast option made by soaking oats overnight with mixed berries for a flavorful morning treat.

Preparation time: 5 minutes

Soaking time: Overnight

Number of servings: 2

Ingredients:

- 1 cup rolled oats

- 1 cup almond milk or any milk of your choice

- 1/2 cup mixed berries (such as strawberries, blueberries, raspberries)

- 2 tablespoons honey or maple syrup

- 1/4 teaspoon vanilla extract

- Optional toppings: sliced almonds, shredded coconut

How to make:

1. In a jar or container, combine rolled oats, almond milk, mixed berries, honey or maple syrup, and vanilla extract.

2. Stir well to mix all ingredients.

3. Cover the jar with a lid and refrigerate overnight.

4. In the morning, give the oats a good stir and add optional toppings if desired.

5. Enjoy cold or warm by heating in the microwave for 1-2 minutes.

Nutritional info: (per serving)

- Calories: 250

- Protein: 6g

- Fat: 4g

- Carbohydrates: 50g

- Fiber: 8g

Chocolate Chia Pudding

Description: A rich and indulgent pudding made with chia seeds and cocoa for a healthy twist on chocolate dessert.

Preparation time: 5 minutes

Chilling time: 2 hours or overnight

Number of servings: 2

Ingredients:

- 1/4 cup chia seeds

- 1 cup almond milk or any milk of your choice

- 2 tablespoons cocoa powder

- 2 tablespoons honey or maple syrup

- 1/2 teaspoon vanilla extract

How to make:

1. In a bowl, whisk together chia seeds, almond milk, cocoa powder, honey or maple syrup, and vanilla extract until well combined.

2. Let the mixture sit for 5 minutes, then whisk
   again to prevent clumps from forming.

3. Cover the bowl and refrigerate for at least 2
   hours or overnight, until the pudding has
   thickened.

4. Stir the pudding before serving and top with
   your favorite toppings if desired.

5. Enjoy cold!

   Nutritional info: (per serving)

- Calories: 200

- Protein: 6g

- Fat: 9g

- Carbohydrates: 25g

- Fiber: 10g

Peanut Butter Overnight Oats

Description: Creamy and satisfying overnight oats flavored with peanut butter for a delicious breakfast option.

Preparation time: 5 minutes

Soaking time: Overnight

Number of servings: 2

Ingredients:

- 1 cup rolled oats

- 1 cup almond milk or any milk of your choice

- 2 tablespoons peanut butter

- 2 tablespoons honey or maple syrup

- Optional toppings: sliced banana, chopped peanuts

How to make:

1. In a jar or container, combine rolled oats, almond milk, peanut butter, and honey or maple syrup.

2. Stir well to mix all ingredients.

3. Cover the jar with a lid and refrigerate overnight.

4. In the morning, give the oats a good stir and add optional toppings if desired.

5. Enjoy cold or warm by heating in the microwave for 1-2 minutes.

Nutritional info: (per serving)

- Calories: 320

- Protein: 10g

- Fat: 12g

- Carbohydrates: 45g

- Fiber: 6g

Mango Coconut Chia Pudding

Description: A tropical twist on classic chia pudding featuring mango and coconut flavors for a refreshing treat.

Preparation time: 5 minutes

Chilling time: 2 hours or overnight

Number of servings: 2

Ingredients:

- 1/4 cup chia seeds

- 1 cup coconut milk

- 1 ripe mango, peeled and diced

- 2 tablespoons honey or maple syrup

- 1/2 teaspoon vanilla extract

How to make:

1. In a bowl, whisk together chia seeds, coconut milk, honey or maple syrup, and vanilla extract until well combined.

2. Gently fold in diced mango.

3. Cover the bowl and refrigerate for at least 2 hours or overnight, until the pudding has thickened.

4. Stir the pudding before serving and top with additional mango or coconut flakes if desired.

5. Enjoy cold!

Nutritional info: (per serving)

- Calories: 250

- Protein: 6g

- Fat: 10g

- Carbohydrates: 35g

- Fiber: 8g

Raspberry Almond Overnight Oats

Description: Nutty and fruity overnight oats flavored with raspberries and almond butter for a delightful breakfast option.

Preparation time: 5 minutes

Soaking time: Overnight

Number of servings: 2

Ingredients:

- 1 cup rolled oats

- 1 cup almond milk or any milk of your choice

- 1/2 cup fresh or frozen raspberries

- 2 tablespoons almond butter

- 2 tablespoons honey or maple syrup

- Optional toppings: sliced almonds, additional raspberries

How to make:

1. In a jar or container, combine rolled oats, almond milk, raspberries, almond butter, and honey or maple syrup.

2. Stir well to mix all ingredients.

3. Cover the jar with a lid and refrigerate overnight.

4. In the morning, give the oats a good stir and
    add optional toppings if desired.

5. Enjoy cold or warm by heating in the
    microwave for 1-2 minutes.

    Nutritional info: (per serving)

- Calories: 300

- Protein: 8g

- Fat: 10g

- Carbohydrates: 45g

- Fiber: 7g

Tofu Scramble with Spinach and Mushrooms

Description: A hearty and flavorful vegan breakfast dish made with tofu, spinach, and mushrooms, seasoned to perfection.

Preparation time: 10 minutes

Cooking time: 15 minutes

Number of servings: 2

Ingredients:

- 1 block (14 oz) firm tofu, drained and crumbled

- 1 cup chopped mushrooms

- 1 cup chopped spinach

- 1/2 onion, finely chopped

- 2 cloves garlic, minced

- 2 tablespoons nutritional yeast

- 1 teaspoon turmeric

- 1/2 teaspoon cumin

- Salt and pepper to taste

- 1 tablespoon olive oil

How to make:

1. Heat olive oil in a skillet over medium heat. Add onions and garlic, sauté until translucent.

2. Add mushrooms and cook until they release their moisture and start to brown.

3. Stir in crumbled tofu, nutritional yeast, turmeric, cumin, salt, and pepper. Cook for 5-7 minutes, stirring occasionally.

4. Add chopped spinach and cook until wilted.

5. Adjust seasoning if necessary and serve hot.

Nutritional info: (per serving)

- Calories: 220

- Protein: 18g

- Fat: 12g

- Carbohydrates: 12g

- Fiber: 5g

Chickpea Flour Omelet

Description: A vegan alternative to traditional omelets made with chickpea flour and filled with your favorite vegetables.

Preparation time: 10 minutes

Cooking time: 10 minutes

Number of servings: 2

Ingredients:

- 1 cup chickpea flour

- 1 cup water

- 1/2 teaspoon baking powder

- Salt and pepper to taste

- 1 cup chopped vegetables (e.g., bell peppers, onions, tomatoes)

- 1 tablespoon olive oil

How to make:

1. In a bowl, whisk together chickpea flour, water, baking powder, salt, and pepper until smooth.

2. Heat olive oil in a non-stick skillet over medium heat.

3. Pour half of the chickpea flour mixture into the skillet, tilting to spread evenly.

4. Cook for 2-3 minutes until the edges start to set.

5. Sprinkle chopped vegetables over one half of the omelet and fold the other half over the filling.

6. Cook for another 2-3 minutes until the omelet is cooked through and golden brown.

7. Repeat with the remaining batter and filling.

8. Serve hot with your favorite sauce or condiments.

Nutritional info: (per serving)

- Calories: 250

- Protein: 12g

- Fat: 10g

- Carbohydrates: 30g

- Fiber: 8g

Southwest Tofu Scramble

Description: A spicy and savory tofu scramble with a southwestern twist, perfect for a hearty breakfast or brunch.

Preparation time: 10 minutes

Cooking time: 15 minutes

Number of servings: 2

Ingredients:

- 1 block (14 oz) firm tofu, drained and crumbled

- 1/2 red bell pepper, diced

- 1/2 green bell pepper, diced

- 1/2 onion, finely chopped

- 1 jalapeño, seeded and diced (optional)

- 2 cloves garlic, minced

- 1 teaspoon chili powder

- 1/2 teaspoon cumin

- Salt and pepper to taste

- 1 tablespoon olive oil

- Fresh cilantro, chopped (for garnish)

How to make:

1. Heat olive oil in a skillet over medium heat. Add onions, garlic, and bell peppers, sauté until softened.

2. Stir in crumbled tofu, jalapeño (if using), chili powder, cumin, salt, and pepper. Cook for 5-7 minutes, stirring occasionally.

3. Adjust seasoning if necessary and serve hot, garnished with chopped cilantro.

Nutritional info: (per serving)

- Calories: 220

- Protein: 18g

- Fat: 10g

- Carbohydrates: 15g

- Fiber: 6g

Vegan Omelet with Roasted Veggies

Description: A flavorful vegan omelet made with a chickpea flour base and filled with roasted vegetables for a satisfying meal.

Preparation time: 15 minutes

Cooking time: 20 minutes

Number of servings: 2

Ingredients:

- 1 cup chickpea flour

- 1 cup water

- 1/2 teaspoon baking powder

- Salt and pepper to taste

- 1 cup roasted vegetables (e.g., bell peppers, zucchini, cherry tomatoes)

- 1 tablespoon olive oil

How to make:

1. In a bowl, whisk together chickpea flour, water, baking powder, salt, and pepper until smooth.

2. Preheat oven to 400°F (200°C). Toss vegetables with olive oil, salt, and pepper, then spread them on a baking sheet.

3. Roast vegetables in the preheated oven for 15-20 minutes, or until tender and slightly caramelized.

4. Heat olive oil in a non-stick skillet over medium heat.

5. Pour half of the chickpea flour mixture into the skillet, tilting to spread evenly.

6. Cook for 2-3 minutes until the edges start to set.

7. Place roasted vegetables over one half of the omelet and fold the other half over the filling.

8. Cook for another 2-3 minutes until the omelet is cooked through and golden brown.

9. Repeat with the remaining batter and filling.

10. Serve hot with your favorite sauce or condiments.

Nutritional info: (per serving)

- Calories: 280

- Protein: 10g

- Fat: 12g

- Carbohydrates: 30g

- Fiber: 8g

Tofu Scramble with Tempeh Bacon

Description: A protein-packed vegan breakfast featuring tofu scramble served alongside savory tempeh bacon for a delicious morning meal.

Preparation time: 10 minutes

Cooking time: 15 minutes

Number of servings: 2

Ingredients:

- 1 block (14 oz) firm tofu, drained and crumbled

- 1 package tempeh bacon

- 1/2 onion, finely chopped

- 2 cloves garlic, minced

- 1 teaspoon smoked paprika

- 1/2 teaspoon turmeric

- Salt and pepper to taste

- 1 tablespoon olive oil

How to make:

1. Heat olive oil in a skillet over medium heat. Add onions and garlic, sauté until translucent.

2. Add crumbled tofu, smoked paprika, turmeric, salt, and pepper. Cook for 5-7 minutes, stirring occasionally.

3. In a separate skillet, cook tempeh bacon
   according to package instructions until
   crispy.

4. Serve tofu scramble and tempeh bacon
   together, garnished with fresh herbs if
   desired.

Nutritional info: (per serving)

- Calories: 300

- Protein: 20g

- Fat: 15g

- Carbohydrates: 20g

- Fiber: 6g

Vegan Banana Pancakes

Description: Fluffy and flavorful pancakes made without eggs or dairy, infused with ripe bananas for a naturally sweet taste.

Preparation time: 10 minutes

Cooking time: 10 minutes

Number of servings: 4

Ingredients:

- 1 cup all-purpose flour

- 1 tablespoon baking powder

- 1/4 teaspoon salt

- 1 ripe banana, mashed

- 1 cup almond milk or any plant-based milk

- 2 tablespoons maple syrup or any sweetener of your choice

- 1 teaspoon vanilla extract

- Optional toppings: sliced bananas, maple syrup, chopped nuts

How to make:

1. In a mixing bowl, whisk together flour, baking powder, and salt.

2. In a separate bowl, mash the ripe banana, then add almond milk, maple syrup, and vanilla extract. Stir until well combined.

3. Pour the wet ingredients into the dry ingredients and mix until just combined. Be careful not to overmix.

4. Heat a non-stick skillet or griddle over medium heat and lightly grease with oil or cooking spray.

5. Pour about 1/4 cup of batter onto the skillet for each pancake.

6. Cook until bubbles form on the surface, then flip and cook until golden brown on both sides.

7. Repeat with the remaining batter.

8. Serve warm with your favorite toppings.

   Nutritional info: (per serving, without toppings)

- Calories: 180

- Protein: 4g

- Fat: 2g

- Carbohydrates: 35g

- Fiber: 2g

Whole Wheat Blueberry Waffles

Description: Nutritious and delicious waffles made with whole wheat flour and bursting with juicy blueberries.

Preparation time: 10 minutes

Cooking time: 10 minutes

Number of servings: 4

Ingredients:

- 1 cup whole wheat flour

- 1 tablespoon baking powder

- 1/4 teaspoon salt

- 1 tablespoon maple syrup or any sweetener of your choice

- 1 cup almond milk or any plant-based milk

- 2 tablespoons melted coconut oil or any vegetable oil

- 1/2 cup fresh or frozen blueberries

- Optional toppings: fresh berries, maple syrup, coconut yogurt

How to make:

1. In a mixing bowl, whisk together whole wheat flour, baking powder, and salt.

2. In a separate bowl, combine maple syrup, almond milk, and melted coconut oil.

3. Pour the wet ingredients into the dry ingredients and mix until just combined.

4. Gently fold in the blueberries.

5. Preheat your waffle iron according to manufacturer's instructions and lightly grease with oil or cooking spray.

6. Pour enough batter onto the waffle iron to cover the grids, then close the lid and cook until golden brown and crispy.

7. Repeat with the remaining batter.

8. Serve warm with your favorite toppings.

   Nutritional info: (per serving, without toppings)

- Calories: 220

- Protein: 5g

- Fat: 7g

- Carbohydrates: 35g

- Fiber: 5g

Cinnamon Raisin French Toast

Description: Classic French toast with a twist, featuring cinnamon and plump raisins for a cozy and comforting breakfast.

Preparation time: 10 minutes

Cooking time: 10 minutes

Number of servings: 4

Ingredients:

- 8 slices whole wheat bread

- 1 cup almond milk or any plant-based milk

- 2 tablespoons maple syrup or any sweetener of your choice

- 1 teaspoon ground cinnamon

- 1 teaspoon vanilla extract

- 1/4 cup raisins

- Coconut oil or vegan butter for cooking

- Optional toppings: maple syrup, powdered sugar, fresh fruit

How to make:

1. In a shallow dish, whisk together almond milk, maple syrup, ground cinnamon, and vanilla extract.

2. Stir in raisins.

3. Dip each slice of bread into the mixture, allowing it to soak for a few seconds on each side.

4. Heat coconut oil or vegan butter in a skillet over medium heat.

5. Cook the soaked bread slices for 3-4 minutes on each side, or until golden brown and crispy.

6. Serve warm with your favorite toppings.

Nutritional info: (per serving, without toppings)

- Calories: 200

- Protein: 5g

- Fat: 3g

- Carbohydrates: 40g

- Fiber: 5g

Lemon Poppyseed Pancakes

Description: Light and fluffy pancakes infused with fresh lemon zest and poppy seeds for a zesty and delightful breakfast.

Preparation time: 10 minutes

Cooking time: 10 minutes

Number of servings: 4

Ingredients:

- 1 cup all-purpose flour

- 1 tablespoon baking powder

- 1/4 teaspoon salt

- Zest of 1 lemon

- 2 tablespoons maple syrup or any sweetener of your choice

- 1 cup almond milk or any plant-based milk

- 2 tablespoons melted coconut oil or any vegetable oil

- 1 tablespoon poppy seeds

- Optional toppings: lemon slices, maple syrup, coconut yogurt

How to make:

1. In a mixing bowl, whisk together all-purpose flour, baking powder, salt, and lemon zest.

2. In a separate bowl, combine maple syrup, almond milk, and melted coconut oil.

3. Pour the wet ingredients into the dry ingredients and mix until just combined.

4. Gently fold in the poppy seeds.

5. Preheat a non-stick skillet or griddle over medium heat and lightly grease with oil or cooking spray.

6. Pour about 1/4 cup of batter onto the skillet for each pancake.

7. Cook until bubbles form on the surface, then flip and cook until golden brown on both sides.

8. Repeat with the remaining batter.

9. Serve warm with your favorite toppings.

   Nutritional info: (per serving, without toppings)

- Calories: 200

- Protein: 4g

- Fat: 7g

- Carbohydrates: 30g

- Fiber: 2g

Sweet Potato Waffles

Description: Nutritious and flavorful waffles made with mashed sweet potatoes for a delightful twist on a breakfast classic.

Preparation time: 15 minutes

Cooking time: 10 minutes

Number of servings: 4

Ingredients:

- 1 cup whole wheat flour

- 1 tablespoon baking powder

- 1/4 teaspoon salt

- 1 cup mashed sweet potatoes (about 1 large sweet potato)

- 1 cup almond milk or any plant-based milk

- 2 tablespoons maple syrup or any sweetener of your choice

- 2 tablespoons melted coconut oil or any vegetable oil

- 1 teaspoon vanilla extract

- Optional toppings: sliced bananas, maple syrup, chopped nuts

How to make:

1. In a mixing bowl, whisk together whole wheat flour, baking powder, and salt.

2. In a separate bowl, combine mashed sweet potatoes, almond milk, maple syrup, melted coconut oil, and vanilla extract.

3. Pour the wet ingredients into the dry ingredients and mix until just combined.

4. Preheat your waffle iron according to manufacturer's instructions and lightly grease with oil or cooking spray.

5. Pour enough batter onto the waffle iron to cover the grids, then close the lid and cook until golden brown and crispy.

6. Repeat with the remaining batter.

7. Serve warm with your favorite toppings.

   Nutritional info: (per serving, without toppings)

- Calories: 250

- Protein: 5g

- Fat: 8g

- Carbohydrates: 40g

- Fiber: 5g

Chocolate Chip Pancakes

Description: Fluffy pancakes studded with chocolate chips for a decadent and indulgent breakfast treat.

Preparation time: 10 minutes

Cooking time: 10 minutes

Number of servings: 4

Ingredients:

- 1 cup all-purpose flour

- 1 tablespoon baking powder

- 1/4 teaspoon salt

- 1 tablespoon sugar

- 1 cup almond milk or any plant-based milk

- 2 tablespoons melted coconut oil or any vegetable oil

- 1 teaspoon vanilla extract

- 1/2 cup vegan chocolate chips

- Optional toppings: maple syrup, additional chocolate chips

How to make:

1. In a mixing bowl, whisk together all-purpose flour, baking powder, salt, and sugar.

2. In a separate bowl, combine almond milk, melted coconut oil, and vanilla extract.

3. Pour the wet ingredients into the dry ingredients and mix until just combined.

4. Gently fold in the vegan chocolate chips.

5. Preheat a non-stick skillet or griddle over medium heat and lightly grease with oil or cooking spray.

6. Pour about 1/4 cup of batter onto the skillet for each pancake.

7. Cook until bubbles form on the surface, then flip and cook until golden brown on both sides.

8. Repeat with the remaining batter.

9. Serve warm with your favorite toppings.

Nutritional info: (per serving, without toppings)

- Calories: 250

- Protein: 4g

- Fat: 10g

- Carbohydrates: 35g

- Fiber: 2g

Buckwheat Waffles with Berry Compote

Description: Nutty and wholesome buckwheat waffles served with a sweet and tangy berry compote for a delightful breakfast.

Preparation time: 15 minutes

Cooking time: 10 minutes

Number of servings: 4

Ingredients:

For the waffles:

- 1 cup buckwheat flour

- 1 tablespoon baking powder

- 1/4 teaspoon salt

- 1 tablespoon sugar

- 1 cup almond milk or any plant-based milk

- 2 tablespoons melted coconut oil or any vegetable oil

- 1 teaspoon vanilla extract

- For the berry compote:

- 2 cups mixed berries (such as strawberries, blueberries, raspberries)

- 2 tablespoons maple syrup or any sweetener of your choice

- Juice of 1/2 lemon

How to make:

1. In a mixing bowl, whisk together buckwheat flour, baking powder, salt, and sugar.

2. In a separate bowl, combine almond milk, melted coconut oil, and vanilla extract.

3. Pour the wet ingredients into the dry ingredients and mix until just combined.

4. Preheat your waffle iron according to manufacturer's instructions and lightly grease with oil or cooking spray.

5. Pour enough batter onto the waffle iron to cover the grids, then close the lid and cook until golden brown and crispy.

6. While the waffles are cooking, prepare the berry compote. In a saucepan, combine mixed berries, maple syrup, and lemon juice.

7. Cook over medium heat, stirring occasionally, until the berries break down and the mixture thickens slightly, about 5-7 minutes.

8. Serve the buckwheat waffles warm with the berry compote.

   Nutritional info: (per serving, waffles only, without toppings)

- Calories: 220

- Protein: 5g

- Fat: 8g

- Carbohydrates: 35g

- Fiber: 5g

Savory Chickpea Flour Pancakes

Description: Flavorful and protein-rich pancakes made with chickpea flour and seasoned with savory herbs and spices.

Preparation time: 10 minutes

Cooking time: 10 minutes

Number of servings: 4

Ingredients:

- 1 cup chickpea flour

- 1 tablespoon nutritional yeast

- 1/2 teaspoon baking powder

- 1/2 teaspoon garlic powder

- 1/2 teaspoon onion powder

- 1/4 teaspoon turmeric

- 1/4 teaspoon salt

- 1 cup water

- 2 tablespoons chopped fresh herbs (such as parsley, chives)

- 2 tablespoons chopped vegetables (such as bell peppers, onions)

- Olive oil for cooking

How to make:

1. In a mixing bowl, whisk together chickpea flour, nutritional yeast, baking powder, garlic powder, onion powder, turmeric, and salt.

2. Gradually add water, stirring until you have a smooth batter.

3. Stir in chopped fresh herbs and vegetables.

4. Heat olive oil in a skillet over medium heat.

5. Pour about 1/4 cup of batter onto the skillet for each pancake.

6. Cook until bubbles form on the surface, then flip and cook until golden brown on both sides.

7. Repeat with the remaining batter.

8. Serve warm with your favorite savory toppings, such as avocado, salsa, or vegan sour cream.

Nutritional info: (per serving, without toppings)

- Calories: 150

- Protein: 7g

- Fat: 5g

- Carbohydrates: 20g

- Fiber: 5g

Vegan French Toast with Caramelized Bananas

Description: A vegan twist on classic French toast, topped with caramelized bananas for a sweet and indulgent breakfast.

Preparation time: 10 minutes

Cooking time: 10 minutes

Number of servings: 4

Ingredients:

- 8 slices whole wheat bread

- 1 cup almond milk or any plant-based milk

- 2 tablespoons maple syrup or any sweetener
  of your choice

- 1 tablespoon ground flaxseeds

- 1 teaspoon ground cinnamon

- 1/2 teaspoon vanilla extract

- Pinch of salt

- 2 ripe bananas, sliced

- 1 tablespoon coconut oil or vegan butter

- Optional toppings: maple syrup, powdered sugar, chopped nuts

How to make:

1. In a shallow dish, whisk together almond milk, maple syrup, ground flaxseeds, cinnamon, vanilla extract, and salt.

2. Heat coconut oil or vegan butter in a skillet over medium heat.

3. Dip each slice of bread into the mixture, allowing it to soak for a few seconds on each side.

4. Cook the soaked bread slices for 3-4 minutes on each side, or until golden brown and crispy.

5. In the same skillet, add sliced bananas and cook until caramelized, about 2-3 minutes per side.

6. Serve the French toast warm, topped with caramelized bananas and your favorite toppings.

   Nutritional info: (per serving, without toppings)

- Calories: 250

- Protein: 5g

- Fat: 8g

- Carbohydrates: 40g

- Fiber: 5g

Pumpkin Spice Waffles

Description: Warm and comforting waffles infused with pumpkin puree and fragrant spices for a cozy fall-inspired breakfast.

Preparation time: 15 minutes

Cooking time: 10 minutes

Number of servings: 4

Ingredients:

- 1 1/2 cups whole wheat flour

- 1 tablespoon baking powder

- 1 teaspoon ground cinnamon

- 1/2 teaspoon ground nutmeg

- 1/4 teaspoon ground ginger

- 1/4 teaspoon ground cloves

- 1/4 teaspoon salt

- 1 cup almond milk or any plant-based milk

- 1/2 cup pumpkin puree

- 1/4 cup maple syrup or any sweetener of your choice

- 2 tablespoons melted coconut oil or any vegetable oil

- 1 teaspoon vanilla extract

- Optional toppings: maple syrup, chopped nuts, whipped coconut cream

How to make:

1. In a mixing bowl, whisk together whole wheat flour, baking powder, ground cinnamon, ground nutmeg, ground ginger, ground cloves, and salt.

2. In a separate bowl, combine almond milk, pumpkin puree, maple syrup, melted coconut oil, and vanilla extract.

3. Pour the wet ingredients into the dry ingredients and mix until just combined.

4. Preheat your waffle iron according to manufacturer's instructions and lightly grease with oil or cooking spray.

5. Pour enough batter onto the waffle iron to cover the grids, then close the lid and cook until golden brown and crispy.

6. Repeat with the remaining batter.

7. Serve warm with your favorite toppings.

   Nutritional info: (per serving, without toppings)

- Calories: 270

- Protein: 5g

- Fat: 8g

- Carbohydrates: 45g

- Fiber: 6g

Chapter 3

Satisfying Salads and Soups

Kale and Quinoa Salad with Lemon Vinaigrette

Description: This vibrant salad combines nutrient-rich kale and protein-packed quinoa, tossed in a zesty lemon vinaigrette.

Preparation time: 15 minutes

Cooking time: 15 minutes

Number of servings: 4

Ingredients:

- 1 bunch kale, stems removed and chopped

- 1 cup quinoa, rinsed

- 2 cups vegetable broth

- 1/4 cup olive oil

- Juice of 1 lemon

- 2 cloves garlic, minced

- Salt and pepper to taste

How to make:

1. In a medium saucepan, bring the vegetable broth to a boil. Add quinoa, reduce heat, cover, and simmer for 15 minutes or until quinoa is cooked and liquid is absorbed. Remove from heat and let it cool.

2. In a small bowl, whisk together olive oil, lemon juice, garlic, salt, and pepper to make the vinaigrette.

3. In a large bowl, massage the kale with a bit of olive oil until it begins to soften.

4. Add cooked quinoa to the kale and toss with lemon vinaigrette until well combined.

5. Serve immediately or refrigerate until ready to serve.

Nutritional info: (per serving)

- Calories: 280

- Protein: 8g

- Fat: 14g

- Carbohydrates: 34g

- Fiber: 4g

Arugula and Wild Rice Salad with Cranberries

Description: A delightful combination of peppery arugula, hearty wild rice, and sweet cranberries, all dressed in a tangy vinaigrette.

Preparation time: 10 minutes

Cooking time: 45 minutes

Number of servings: 4

Ingredients:

- 1 cup wild rice
- 4 cups arugula
- 1/2 cup dried cranberries

- 1/4 cup sliced almonds

- 2 tablespoons balsamic vinegar

- 1 tablespoon honey

- 2 tablespoons olive oil

- Salt and pepper to taste

How to make:

1. Cook wild rice according to package instructions. Once cooked, let it cool to room temperature.

2. In a small bowl, whisk together balsamic vinegar, honey, olive oil, salt, and pepper to make the dressing.

3. In a large bowl, combine cooked wild rice, arugula, dried cranberries, and sliced almonds.

4. Drizzle the dressing over the salad and toss until everything is well coated.

5. Serve immediately or refrigerate until ready to serve.

Nutritional info: (per serving)

- Calories: 320

- Protein: 7g

- Fat: 10g

- Carbohydrates: 52g

- Fiber: 5g

Mediterranean Farro Salad

Description: A hearty salad featuring nutty farro, crisp vegetables, briny olives, and tangy feta cheese, all tossed in a lemony dressing.

Preparation time: 20 minutes

Cooking time: 30 minutes

Number of servings: 6

Ingredients:

- 1 cup farro

- 2 cups water or vegetable broth

- 1 cup cherry tomatoes, halved

- 1 cucumber, diced

- 1/2 cup Kalamata olives, sliced

- 1/4 cup red onion, thinly sliced

- 1/2 cup crumbled feta cheese

- 1/4 cup chopped fresh parsley

- Juice of 1 lemon

- 2 tablespoons extra virgin olive oil

- Salt and pepper to taste

How to make:

1. In a medium saucepan, bring water or vegetable broth to a boil. Add farro, reduce heat, cover, and simmer for 30 minutes or until farro is tender. Drain any excess liquid and let it cool.

2. In a large bowl, combine cooked farro, cherry tomatoes, cucumber, olives, red onion, feta cheese, and parsley.

3. In a small bowl, whisk together lemon juice, olive oil, salt, and pepper to make the dressing.

4. Drizzle the dressing over the salad and toss until everything is well coated.

5. Serve immediately or refrigerate until ready to serve.

Nutritional info: (per serving)

- Calories: 280

- Protein: 7g

- Fat: 8g

- Carbohydrates: 45g

- Fiber: 7g

Spinach and Buckwheat Salad with Roasted Beets

Description: A wholesome salad featuring earthy spinach, nutty buckwheat, sweet roasted beets, and creamy goat cheese, all tossed in a balsamic vinaigrette.

Preparation time: 15 minutes

Cooking time: 45 minutes

Number of servings: 4

Ingredients:

- 1 cup buckwheat groats

- 2 cups water or vegetable broth

- 2 cups baby spinach

- 2 medium beets, roasted and diced

- 1/4 cup crumbled goat cheese

- 2 tablespoons balsamic vinegar

- 1 tablespoon maple syrup

- 2 tablespoons extra virgin olive oil

- Salt and pepper to taste

How to make:

1. In a medium saucepan, bring water or vegetable broth to a boil. Add buckwheat groats, reduce heat, cover, and simmer for 15 minutes or until buckwheat is tender. Drain any excess liquid and let it cool.

2. In a large bowl, combine cooked buckwheat, baby spinach, roasted beets, and crumbled goat cheese.

3. In a small bowl, whisk together balsamic vinegar, maple syrup, olive oil, salt, and pepper to make the dressing.

4. Drizzle the dressing over the salad and toss until everything is well coated.

5. Serve immediately or refrigerate until ready
    to serve.

Nutritional info: (per serving)

- Calories: 320

- Protein: 8g

- Fat: 10g

- Carbohydrates: 50g

- Fiber: 7g

Massaged Kale Salad with Apple and Pecans

Description: A refreshing salad featuring massaged kale, crisp apple slices, crunchy pecans, and a sweet and tangy maple vinaigrette.

Preparation time: 10 minutes

Cooking time: 0 minutes

Number of servings: 4

Ingredients:

- 1 bunch kale, stems removed and chopped

- 1 apple, thinly sliced

- 1/2 cup chopped pecans

- 1/4 cup dried cranberries

- 2 tablespoons apple cider vinegar

- 1 tablespoon maple syrup

- 2 tablespoons olive oil

- Salt and pepper to taste

How to make:

1. In a large bowl, combine kale, apple slices, chopped pecans, and dried cranberries.

2. In a small bowl, whisk together apple cider vinegar, maple syrup, olive oil, salt, and pepper to make the dressing.

3. Pour the dressing over the salad and massage it into the kale leaves for a few minutes until they begin to soften.

4. Serve immediately or refrigerate until ready to serve.

Nutritional info: (per serving)

- Calories: 240

- Protein: 4g

- Fat: 14g

- Carbohydrates: 28g

- Fiber: 4g

Three Bean Salad with Herb Vinaigrette

Description: A classic salad featuring a trio of beans (kidney beans, green beans, and wax beans) tossed in a flavorful herb vinaigrette.

Preparation time: 15 minutes

Cooking time: 5 minutes

Number of servings: 6

Ingredients:

- 1 can (15 oz) kidney beans, drained and rinsed

- 1 can (15 oz) green beans, drained and rinsed

- 1 can (15 oz) wax beans, drained and rinsed

- 1/4 cup red onion, finely chopped

- 1/4 cup fresh parsley, chopped

- 2 tablespoons fresh dill, chopped

- 2 tablespoons apple cider vinegar

- 2 tablespoons olive oil

- 1 teaspoon Dijon mustard

- Salt and pepper to taste

How to make:

1. In a large bowl, combine kidney beans, green beans, wax beans, red onion, parsley, and dill.

2. In a small bowl, whisk together apple cider vinegar, olive oil, Dijon mustard, salt, and pepper to make the vinaigrette.

3. Pour the vinaigrette over the bean mixture and toss until well combined.

4. Serve immediately or refrigerate until ready to serve.

Nutritional info: (per serving)

- Calories: 180

- Protein: 7g

- Fat: 5g

- Carbohydrates: 28g

- Fiber: 8g

Lentil and Roasted Vegetable Salad

Description: A hearty salad featuring protein-rich lentils and roasted vegetables, all tossed in a savory dressing.

Preparation time: 15 minutes

Cooking time: 30 minutes

Number of servings: 4

Ingredients:

- 1 cup green or brown lentils, rinsed

- 2 cups water or vegetable broth

- 2 cups mixed vegetables (such as bell peppers, zucchini, and carrots), diced

- 2 tablespoons olive oil

- 2 cloves garlic, minced

- 1 teaspoon dried thyme

- Salt and pepper to taste

- 2 tablespoons balsamic vinegar

How to make:

1. In a medium saucepan, bring water or vegetable broth to a boil. Add lentils, reduce heat, cover, and simmer for 20-25 minutes or until lentils are tender. Drain any excess liquid and let them cool.

2. Preheat the oven to 400°F (200°C). Place diced vegetables on a baking sheet, drizzle with olive oil, garlic, thyme, salt, and pepper. Toss to coat evenly. Roast for 20-25 minutes or until vegetables are tender and lightly browned.

3. In a large bowl, combine cooked lentils and roasted vegetables.

4. Drizzle balsamic vinegar over the salad and toss until everything is well coated.

5. Serve immediately or refrigerate until ready to serve.

Nutritional info: (per serving)

- Calories: 280

- Protein: 12g

- Fat: 7g

- Carbohydrates: 42g

- Fiber: 15g

Black Bean and Mango Salad

Description: A refreshing salad featuring black beans, sweet mango chunks, crisp vegetables, and a tangy lime dressing.

Preparation time: 15 minutes

Cooking time: 0 minutes

Number of servings: 4

Ingredients:

- 1 can (15 oz) black beans, drained and rinsed

- 1 ripe mango, peeled and diced

- 1 red bell pepper, diced

- 1/2 red onion, finely chopped

- 1/4 cup fresh cilantro, chopped

- Juice of 2 limes

- 2 tablespoons olive oil

- 1 teaspoon honey or agave syrup

- Salt and pepper to taste

How to make:

1. In a large bowl, combine black beans, diced mango, red bell pepper, red onion, and cilantro.

2. In a small bowl, whisk together lime juice, olive oil, honey, salt, and pepper to make the dressing.

3. Pour the dressing over the salad and toss until everything is well coated.

4. Serve immediately or refrigerate until ready to serve.

Nutritional info: (per serving)

- Calories: 260

- Protein: 9g

- Fat: 7g

- Carbohydrates: 42g

- Fiber: 11g

White Bean and Arugula Salad with Lemon Dressing

Description: A light and flavorful salad featuring creamy white beans, peppery arugula, and a zesty lemon dressing.

Preparation time: 10 minutes

Cooking time: 0 minutes

Number of servings: 4

Ingredients:

- 1 can (15 oz) cannellini beans, drained and rinsed

- 4 cups arugula

- 1/4 cup grated Parmesan cheese (optional)

- Juice of 1 lemon

- 2 tablespoons extra virgin olive oil

- 1 teaspoon Dijon mustard

- Salt and pepper to taste

How to make:

1. In a large bowl, combine cannellini beans and arugula. If using, sprinkle grated Parmesan cheese on top.

2. In a small bowl, whisk together lemon juice, olive oil, Dijon mustard, salt, and pepper to make the dressing.

3. Pour the dressing over the salad and toss until everything is well coated.

4. Serve immediately or refrigerate until ready to serve.

Nutritional info: (per serving)

- Calories: 220

- Protein: 9g

- Fat: 7g

- Carbohydrates: 30g

- Fiber: 8g

Chickpea Salad with Avocado and Feta

Description: A creamy and satisfying salad featuring protein-packed chickpeas, creamy avocado, tangy feta cheese, and a refreshing lemon dressing.

Preparation time: 15 minutes

Cooking time: 0 minutes

Number of servings: 4

Ingredients:

- 1 can (15 oz) chickpeas, drained and rinsed

- 1 avocado, diced

- 1/4 cup crumbled feta cheese

- 1/4 cup diced red onion

- 1/4 cup chopped fresh parsley

- Juice of 1 lemon

- 2 tablespoons extra virgin olive oil

- Salt and pepper to taste

How to make:

1. In a large bowl, combine chickpeas, diced avocado, crumbled feta cheese, red onion, and parsley.

2. In a small bowl, whisk together lemon juice, olive oil, salt, and pepper to make the dressing.

3. Pour the dressing over the salad and toss until everything is well coated.

4. Serve immediately or refrigerate until ready to serve.

Nutritional info: (per serving)

- Calories: 290

- Protein: 9g

- Fat: 16g

- Carbohydrates: 29g

- Fiber: 10g

Gazpacho (Chilled Tomato Soup)

Description: A refreshing and flavorful chilled soup made with ripe tomatoes, cucumbers, bell peppers, onions, garlic, and a blend of herbs and spices.

Preparation time: 20 minutes

Chilling time: 2 hours

Number of servings: 4

Ingredients:

- 4 large tomatoes, diced
- 1 cucumber, peeled and diced

- 1 bell pepper, diced

- 1/2 red onion, diced

- 2 cloves garlic, minced

- 2 tablespoons olive oil

- 2 tablespoons red wine vinegar

- 1 teaspoon Worcestershire sauce

- Salt and pepper to taste

- 1/4 cup fresh basil leaves, chopped

- Croutons and chopped fresh herbs for garnish (optional)

How to make:

1. In a blender or food processor, combine tomatoes, cucumber, bell pepper, red onion, garlic, olive oil, red wine vinegar,

Worcestershire sauce, salt, and pepper. Blend until smooth.

2. Taste and adjust seasoning if needed. If the soup is too thick, you can add a little water to reach your desired consistency.

3. Transfer the soup to a large bowl, cover, and refrigerate for at least 2 hours to chill.

4. Before serving, stir in chopped basil leaves. Serve chilled, garnished with croutons and chopped fresh herbs if desired.

Nutritional info: (per serving)

- Calories: 120

- Protein: 2g

- Fat: 7g

- Carbohydrates: 14g

- Fiber: 4g

Chilled Cucumber and Avocado Soup

Description: A creamy and refreshing chilled soup made with cool cucumbers, creamy avocado, yogurt, and a hint of lemon.

Preparation time: 10 minutes

Chilling time: 1 hour

Number of servings: 4

Ingredients:

- 2 cucumbers, peeled and chopped

- 1 ripe avocado, peeled and diced

- 1 cup plain yogurt

- Juice of 1 lemon

- 2 tablespoons fresh dill, chopped

- Salt and pepper to taste

- Chopped fresh herbs for garnish (optional)

How to make:

1. In a blender or food processor, combine chopped cucumbers, diced avocado, yogurt, lemon juice, dill, salt, and pepper. Blend until smooth.

2. Taste and adjust seasoning if needed.

3. Transfer the soup to a large bowl, cover, and refrigerate for at least 1 hour to chill.

4. Before serving, stir the soup well. Garnish with chopped fresh herbs if desired.

Nutritional info: (per serving)

- Calories: 150

- Protein: 5g

- Fat: 10g

- Carbohydrates: 12g

- Fiber: 6g

Watermelon Gazpacho

Description: A light and refreshing chilled soup made with juicy watermelon, cucumbers, bell peppers, tomatoes, and a hint of lime.

Preparation time: 15 minutes

Chilling time: 2 hours

Number of servings: 4

Ingredients:

- 4 cups seedless watermelon, chopped

- 1 cucumber, peeled and chopped

- 1 red bell pepper, chopped

- 1 tomato, chopped

- 1/4 cup red onion, chopped

- Juice of 2 limes

- 2 tablespoons fresh mint leaves, chopped

- Salt and pepper to taste

- Crumbled feta cheese for garnish (optional)

How to make:

1. In a blender or food processor, combine chopped watermelon, cucumber, bell pepper, tomato, red onion, lime juice, mint leaves, salt, and pepper. Blend until smooth.

2. Taste and adjust seasoning if needed.

3. Transfer the soup to a large bowl, cover, and refrigerate for at least 2 hours to chill.

4. Before serving, stir the soup well. Serve chilled, garnished with crumbled feta cheese if desired.

Nutritional info: (per serving)

- Calories: 90

- Protein: 2g

- Fat: 1g

- Carbohydrates: 22g

- Fiber: 3g

Chilled Beet and Yogurt Soup

Description: A vibrant and creamy chilled soup made with roasted beets, Greek yogurt, garlic, and a touch of lemon.

Preparation time: 15 minutes

Cooking time: 45 minutes (for roasting beets)

Chilling time: 2 hours

Number of servings: 4

Ingredients:

- 3 medium beets, roasted, peeled, and chopped

- 1 cup plain Greek yogurt

- 2 cloves garlic, minced

- Juice of 1 lemon

- 2 cups vegetable broth

- Salt and pepper to taste

- Chopped fresh dill for garnish (optional)

How to make:

1. In a blender or food processor, combine roasted beets, Greek yogurt, minced garlic, lemon juice, vegetable broth, salt, and pepper. Blend until smooth.

2. Taste and adjust seasoning if needed.

3. Transfer the soup to a large bowl, cover, and refrigerate for at least 2 hours to chill.

4. Before serving, stir the soup well. Garnish with chopped fresh dill if desired.

Nutritional info: (per serving)

- Calories: 100

- Protein: 7g

- Fat: 1g

- Carbohydrates: 17g

- Fiber: 4g

Chilled Cantaloupe Soup with Mint

Description: A refreshing and fragrant chilled soup made with ripe cantaloupe, Greek yogurt, fresh mint, and a hint of honey.

Preparation time: 10 minutes

Chilling time: 1 hour

Number of servings: 4

Ingredients:

- 1 ripe cantaloupe, peeled, seeded, and chopped

- 1 cup plain Greek yogurt

- 2 tablespoons fresh mint leaves, chopped

- 1 tablespoon honey

- Juice of 1 lime

- Pinch of salt

- Fresh mint leaves for garnish (optional)

How to make:

1. In a blender or food processor, combine chopped cantaloupe, Greek yogurt, chopped mint leaves, honey, lime juice, and a pinch of salt. Blend until smooth.

2. Taste and adjust sweetness if needed by adding more honey.

3. Transfer the soup to a large bowl, cover, and refrigerate for at least 1 hour to chill.

4. Before serving, stir the soup well. Garnish with fresh mint leaves if desired.

Nutritional info: (per serving)

- Calories: 100

- Protein: 5g

- Fat: 1g

- Carbohydrates: 22g

- Fiber: 2g

Lentil and Sweet Potato Soup

Description: A hearty and nutritious soup featuring protein-rich lentils, sweet potatoes, carrots, and warming spices.

Preparation time: 15 minutes

Cooking time: 30 minutes

Number of servings: 6

Ingredients:

- 1 cup dried brown lentils, rinsed

- 2 sweet potatoes, peeled and diced

- 2 carrots, peeled and chopped

- 1 onion, chopped

- 2 cloves garlic, minced

- 1 teaspoon ground cumin

- 1/2 teaspoon ground turmeric

- 1/2 teaspoon ground cinnamon

- 6 cups vegetable broth

- Salt and pepper to taste

- Fresh cilantro or parsley for garnish (optional)

How to make:

1. In a large pot, heat some oil over medium heat. Add the onion and garlic, and cook until softened, about 5 minutes.

2. Stir in the lentils, sweet potatoes, carrots, cumin, turmeric, cinnamon, vegetable broth, salt, and pepper.

3. Bring the mixture to a boil, then reduce the heat to low, cover, and simmer for 25-30 minutes, or until the lentils and vegetables are tender.

4. Taste and adjust seasoning if necessary. Serve hot, garnished with fresh cilantro or parsley if desired.

Nutritional info: (per serving)

- Calories: 220

- Protein: 12g

- Fat: 1g

- Carbohydrates: 44g

- Fiber: 12g

Vegan Minestrone Soup

Description: A comforting and hearty soup filled with vegetables, beans, and pasta in a flavorful tomato broth.

Preparation time: 15 minutes

Cooking time: 30 minutes

Number of servings: 6

Ingredients:

- 1 tablespoon olive oil

- 1 onion, chopped

- 2 carrots, diced

- 2 celery stalks, diced

- 3 cloves garlic, minced

- 1 can (15 oz) diced tomatoes

- 6 cups vegetable broth

- 1 can (15 oz) kidney beans, drained and rinsed

- 1 cup small pasta (such as elbow or ditalini)

- 2 cups chopped spinach or kale

- 1 teaspoon dried oregano

- 1 teaspoon dried basil

- Salt and pepper to taste

- Vegan parmesan cheese for garnish (optional)

How to make:

1. In a large pot, heat olive oil over medium heat. Add the onion, carrots, and celery, and cook until softened, about 5 minutes.

2. Stir in the garlic and cook for another minute.

3. Add the diced tomatoes, vegetable broth, kidney beans, pasta, oregano, basil, salt, and pepper. Bring to a simmer and cook for 10-15 minutes, or until the pasta is tender.

4. Stir in the chopped spinach or kale and cook for another 2-3 minutes until wilted.

5. Taste and adjust seasoning if necessary. Serve hot, garnished with vegan parmesan cheese if desired.

Nutritional info: (per serving)

- Calories: 280

- Protein: 10g

- Fat: 3g

- Carbohydrates: 52g

- Fiber: 11g

Creamy Broccoli Soup

Description: A velvety smooth and creamy soup made with tender broccoli florets, onions, garlic, and vegetable broth.

Preparation time: 10 minutes

Cooking time: 25 minutes

Number of servings: 4

Ingredients:

- 2 tablespoons olive oil

- 1 onion, chopped

- 2 cloves garlic, minced

- 4 cups broccoli florets

- 4 cups vegetable broth

- 1/2 cup coconut milk or cashew cream

- Salt and pepper to taste

- Squeeze of lemon juice (optional)

- Toasted pumpkin seeds or croutons for garnish (optional)

How to make:

1. In a large pot, heat olive oil over medium heat. Add the chopped onion and garlic, and cook until softened, about 5 minutes.

2. Add the broccoli florets and vegetable broth to the pot. Bring to a boil, then reduce the heat and simmer for 15-20 minutes, or until the broccoli is tender.

3. Using an immersion blender or transferring the soup to a blender, blend until smooth and creamy.

4. Stir in the coconut milk or cashew cream, and season with salt and pepper to taste. Add a squeeze of lemon juice if desired.

5. Serve hot, garnished with toasted pumpkin seeds or croutons if desired.

Nutritional info: (per serving)

- Calories: 180

- Protein: 5g

- Fat: 12g

- Carbohydrates: 15g

- Fiber: 5g

Spicy Black Bean Soup

Description: A flavorful and satisfying soup made with black beans, vegetables, and a blend of spices for a kick of heat.

Preparation time: 10 minutes

Cooking time: 25 minutes

Number of servings: 4

Ingredients:

- 2 tablespoons olive oil

- 1 onion, chopped

- 2 cloves garlic, minced

- 1 red bell pepper, chopped

- 1 jalapeno pepper, seeded and minced

- 2 teaspoons ground cumin

- 1 teaspoon chili powder

- 1/2 teaspoon smoked paprika

- 2 cans (15 oz each) black beans, drained and rinsed

- 4 cups vegetable broth

- Juice of 1 lime

- Salt and pepper to taste

- Chopped fresh cilantro for garnish (optional)

How to make:

1. In a large pot, heat olive oil over medium heat. Add the chopped onion, garlic, red bell pepper, and jalapeno pepper. Cook until softened, about 5 minutes.

2. Stir in the ground cumin, chili powder, and smoked paprika, and cook for another minute until fragrant.

3. Add the black beans and vegetable broth to the pot. Bring to a boil, then reduce the heat and simmer for 15-20 minutes.

4. Using an immersion blender or transferring the soup to a blender, blend until smooth (you can also leave some beans whole for texture if desired).

5. Stir in the lime juice, and season with salt and pepper to taste.

6. Serve hot, garnished with chopped fresh cilantro if desired.

Nutritional info: (per serving)

- Calories: 280

- Protein: 13g

- Fat: 7g

- Carbohydrates: 45g

- Fiber: 14g

Butternut Squash and Red Lentil Soup

Description: A velvety smooth and comforting soup made with roasted butternut squash, red lentils, onions, garlic, and warming spices.

Preparation time: 15 minutes

Cooking time: 45 minutes

Number of servings: 6

Ingredients:

- 1 medium butternut squash, peeled, seeded, and diced

- 1 onion, chopped

- 2 cloves garlic, minced

- 1 cup red lentils, rinsed

- 6 cups vegetable broth

- 1 teaspoon ground cumin

- 1/2 teaspoon ground coriander

- 1/2 teaspoon ground cinnamon

- Salt and pepper to taste

- Coconut milk or cashew cream for garnish (optional)

How to make:

1. Preheat the oven to 400°F (200°C). Place diced butternut squash on a baking sheet,

drizzle with olive oil, and season with salt and pepper. Roast for 25-30 minutes, or until tender and caramelized.

2. In a large pot, heat some olive oil over medium heat. Add the chopped onion and garlic, and cook until softened, about 5 minutes.

3. Add the roasted butternut squash, red lentils, vegetable broth, ground cumin, ground coriander, and ground cinnamon to the pot. Bring to a boil, then reduce the heat and simmer for 20-25 minutes, or until the lentils are cooked through.

4. Using an immersion blender or transferring the soup to a blender, blend until smooth and creamy.

5. Taste and adjust seasoning if necessary. Serve hot, garnished with a swirl of coconut milk or cashew cream if desired.

Nutritional info: (per serving)

- Calories: 220

- Protein: 10g

- Fat: 1g

- Carbohydrates: 42g

- Fiber: 10g

Vegetable Barley Soup

Description: A comforting and hearty soup made with tender barley, a variety of vegetables, and savory broth.

Preparation time: 15 minutes

Cooking time: 45 minutes

Number of servings: 6

Ingredients:

- 1 tablespoon olive oil

- 1 onion, chopped

- 2 carrots, diced

- 2 celery stalks, diced

- 2 cloves garlic, minced

- 1 cup pearl barley

- 6 cups vegetable broth

- 2 cups chopped mixed vegetables (such as green beans, peas, corn)

- Salt and pepper to taste

- Fresh parsley for garnish (optional)

How to make:

1. In a large pot, heat olive oil over medium heat. Add the chopped onion, carrots, celery, and garlic, and cook until softened, about 5 minutes.

2. Stir in the pearl barley and vegetable broth. Bring to a boil, then reduce the heat and simmer for 30 minutes.

3. Add the chopped mixed vegetables to the pot and simmer for another 10-15 minutes, or until the barley and vegetables are tender.

4. Season with salt and pepper to taste. Serve hot, garnished with fresh parsley if desired.

Nutritional info: (per serving)

- Calories: 250

- Protein: 6g

- Fat: 3g

- Carbohydrates: 52g

- Fiber: 10g

Curried Cauliflower Soup

Description: A creamy and aromatic soup made with roasted cauliflower, onions, garlic, and a blend of curry spices.

Preparation time: 15 minutes

Cooking time: 30 minutes

Number of servings: 4

Ingredients:

- 1 large head cauliflower, chopped into florets

- 2 tablespoons olive oil

- 1 onion, chopped

- 2 cloves garlic, minced

- 1 tablespoon curry powder

- 1 teaspoon ground cumin

- 4 cups vegetable broth

- 1 cup coconut milk

- Salt and pepper to taste

- Fresh cilantro for garnish (optional)

How to make:

1. Preheat the oven to 400°F (200°C). Place cauliflower florets on a baking sheet, drizzle with olive oil, and season with salt and

pepper. Roast for 25-30 minutes, or until tender and golden brown.

2. In a large pot, heat some olive oil over medium heat. Add the chopped onion and garlic, and cook until softened, about 5 minutes.

3. Stir in the curry powder and ground cumin, and cook for another minute until fragrant.

4. Add the roasted cauliflower and vegetable broth to the pot. Bring to a simmer and cook for 15-20 minutes.

5. Using an immersion blender or transferring the soup to a blender, blend until smooth.

6. Stir in the coconut milk, and season with salt and pepper to taste.

7. Serve hot, garnished with fresh cilantro if desired.

Nutritional info: (per serving)

- Calories: 220

- Protein: 5g

- Fat: 16g

- Carbohydrates: 18g

- Fiber: 5g

Tomato and White Bean Soup

Description: A comforting and flavorful soup made with juicy tomatoes, creamy white beans, onions, garlic, and Italian herbs.

Preparation time: 10 minutes

Cooking time: 25 minutes

Number of servings: 4

Ingredients:

- 1 tablespoon olive oil

- 1 onion, chopped

- 2 cloves garlic, minced

- 1 can (15 oz) diced tomatoes

- 2 cups vegetable broth

- 1 can (15 oz) white beans, drained and rinsed

- 1 teaspoon dried basil

- 1 teaspoon dried oregano

- Salt and pepper to taste

- Fresh basil for garnish (optional)

How to make:

1. In a large pot, heat olive oil over medium heat. Add the chopped onion and garlic, and cook until softened, about 5 minutes.

2. Stir in the diced tomatoes (with their juices), vegetable broth, white beans, dried basil, dried oregano, salt, and pepper. Bring to a simmer and cook for 15-20 minutes.

3. Using an immersion blender or transferring the soup to a blender, blend a portion of the soup until smooth (optional for a creamier texture).

4. Taste and adjust seasoning if necessary. Serve hot, garnished with fresh basil if desired.

Nutritional info: (per serving)

- Calories: 180

- Protein: 8g

- Fat: 3g

- Carbohydrates: 30g

- Fiber: 8g

Coconut Curry Lentil Soup

Description: A creamy and flavorful soup made with red lentils, coconut milk, tomatoes, onions, garlic, and a blend of curry spices.

Preparation time: 10 minutes

Cooking time: 25 minutes

Number of servings: 4

Ingredients:

- 1 tablespoon coconut oil

- 1 onion, chopped

- 2 cloves garlic, minced

- 1 tablespoon curry powder

- 1 teaspoon ground cumin

- 1 cup red lentils, rinsed

- 1 can (15 oz) diced tomatoes

- 4 cups vegetable broth

- 1 cup coconut milk

- Salt and pepper to taste

- Fresh cilantro for garnish (optional)

How to make:

1. In a large pot, heat coconut oil over medium heat. Add the chopped onion and garlic, and cook until softened, about 5 minutes.

2. Stir in the curry powder and ground cumin, and cook for another minute until fragrant.

3. Add the red lentils, diced tomatoes (with their juices), and vegetable broth to the pot. Bring to a simmer and cook for 15-20 minutes, or until the lentils are tender.

4. Stir in the coconut milk, and season with salt and pepper to taste.

5. Serve hot, garnished with fresh cilantro if desired.

Nutritional info: (per serving)

- Calories: 340

- Protein: 13g

- Fat: 15g

- Carbohydrates: 41g

- Fiber: 16g

Roasted Garlic and Potato Soup

Description: A creamy and comforting soup made with roasted garlic, potatoes, onions, and savory broth.

Preparation time: 15 minutes

Cooking time: 45 minutes

Number of servings: 4

Ingredients:

- 1 head garlic

- 1 tablespoon olive oil

- 1 onion, chopped

- 2 large potatoes, peeled and diced

- 4 cups vegetable broth

- 1/2 cup coconut milk or cashew cream

- Salt and pepper to taste

- Fresh chives for garnish (optional)

How to make:

1. Preheat the oven to 400°F (200°C). Slice off the top of the head of garlic to expose the cloves. Drizzle with olive oil, wrap in aluminum foil, and roast for 30-35 minutes, or until soft and caramelized.

2. In a large pot, heat some olive oil over medium heat. Add the chopped onion and cook until softened, about 5 minutes.

3. Add the diced potatoes and vegetable broth to the pot. Bring to a boil, then reduce the heat and simmer for 15-20 minutes, or until the potatoes are tender.

4. Squeeze the roasted garlic cloves out of their skins and add them to the pot.

5. Using an immersion blender or transferring the soup to a blender, blend until smooth and creamy.

6. Stir in the coconut milk or cashew cream, and season with salt and pepper to taste.

7. Serve hot, garnished with fresh chives if desired.

Nutritional info: (per serving)

216

- Calories: 220

- Protein: 5g

- Fat: 6g

- Carbohydrates: 38g

- Fiber: 5g

Chapter 4

Plant-Powered Mains

Tofu and Vegetable Stir-Fry with Peanut Sauce

Description: A flavorful stir-fry featuring tofu and a variety of vegetables, all coated in a rich and creamy peanut sauce.

Preparation time: 15 minutes

Cooking time: 15 minutes

Number of servings: 4

Ingredients:

- 14 oz (400g) firm tofu, drained and cubed

- 2 cups mixed vegetables (such as bell peppers, broccoli, carrots, and snow peas), chopped

- 2 cloves garlic, minced

- 1 tablespoon ginger, minced

- 2 tablespoons soy sauce

- 3 tablespoons peanut butter

- 2 tablespoons water

- 1 tablespoon sesame oil

- 1 tablespoon vegetable oil

- Salt and pepper to taste

- Cooked rice or noodles, for serving

- Crushed peanuts and chopped cilantro, for garnish (optional)

How to make:

1. In a small bowl, mix together soy sauce, peanut butter, and water to make the peanut sauce. Set aside.

2. Heat vegetable oil in a large skillet or wok over medium-high heat. Add tofu cubes and cook until golden brown on all sides, about 5-7 minutes. Remove tofu from the skillet and set aside.

3. In the same skillet, add sesame oil, garlic, and ginger. Cook for 1-2 minutes until fragrant.

4. Add mixed vegetables to the skillet and stir-fry for 3-5 minutes until they are tender but still crisp.

5. Return the tofu to the skillet and pour the peanut sauce over the tofu and vegetables. Stir well to coat everything evenly.

6. Cook for an additional 2-3 minutes, stirring constantly, until the sauce is heated through and the tofu and vegetables are well coated.

7. Season with salt and pepper to taste.

8. Serve the stir-fry hot over cooked rice or noodles, garnished with crushed peanuts and chopped cilantro if desired.

Nutritional info: (per serving)

- Calories: 320

- Fat: 20g

- Carbohydrates: 20g

- Protein: 18g

Cashew Vegetable Stir-Fry

Description: A delightful stir-fry packed with colorful vegetables and crunchy cashews, seasoned to perfection.

Preparation time: 15 minutes

Cooking time: 15 minutes

Number of servings: 4

Ingredients:

- 2 cups mixed vegetables (such as bell peppers, broccoli, carrots, and snap peas), chopped
- 1 cup cashews

- 2 cloves garlic, minced

- 1 tablespoon ginger, minced

- 3 tablespoons soy sauce

- 1 tablespoon rice vinegar

- 1 tablespoon hoisin sauce

- 1 tablespoon sesame oil

- 1 tablespoon vegetable oil

- Cooked rice or noodles, for serving

How to make:

1. Heat vegetable oil in a large skillet or wok over medium-high heat.

2. Add garlic and ginger to the skillet and cook for 1-2 minutes until fragrant.

3. Add mixed vegetables to the skillet and stir-fry for 3-5 minutes until they are tender but still crisp.

4. In a small bowl, whisk together soy sauce, rice vinegar, and hoisin sauce.

5. Pour the sauce over the vegetables in the skillet and stir well to coat.

6. Add cashews to the skillet and continue to cook for an additional 2-3 minutes, stirring constantly.

7. Drizzle sesame oil over the stir-fry and toss to combine.

8. Serve the stir-fry hot over cooked rice or noodles.

Nutritional info: (per serving)

- Calories: 280

- Fat: 18g

- Carbohydrates: 22g

- Protein: 10g

Teriyaki Vegetable Stir-Fry

Description: A savory stir-fry featuring a medley of vegetables tossed in a homemade teriyaki sauce.

Preparation time: 15 minutes

Cooking time: 15 minutes

Number of servings: 4

Ingredients:

- 2 cups mixed vegetables (such as bell peppers, mushrooms, onions, and broccoli), chopped

- 1 cup tofu or chicken, diced (optional)

- 2 cloves garlic, minced

- 1 tablespoon ginger, minced

- 3 tablespoons soy sauce

- 2 tablespoons honey

- 1 tablespoon rice vinegar

- 1 tablespoon cornstarch

- 1 tablespoon vegetable oil

- Cooked rice or noodles, for serving

How to make:

1. In a small bowl, whisk together soy sauce, honey, rice vinegar, and cornstarch to make the teriyaki sauce. Set aside.

2. Heat vegetable oil in a large skillet or wok over medium-high heat.

3. Add garlic and ginger to the skillet and cook for 1-2 minutes until fragrant.

4. If using tofu or chicken, add it to the skillet and cook until browned on all sides, about 5-7 minutes. Remove from the skillet and set aside.

5. Add mixed vegetables to the skillet and stir-fry for 3-5 minutes until they are tender but still crisp.

6. Return tofu or chicken to the skillet (if using) and pour the teriyaki sauce over the

vegetables. Stir well to coat everything evenly.

7. Cook for an additional 2-3 minutes, stirring constantly, until the sauce has thickened and the tofu or chicken is heated through.

8. Serve the stir-fry hot over cooked rice or noodles.

Nutritional info: (per serving)

- Calories: 250

- Fat: 6g

- Carbohydrates: 35g

- Protein: 12g

Szechuan Eggplant and Broccoli Stir-Fry

Description: A spicy and aromatic stir-fry featuring tender eggplant and crisp broccoli, seasoned with bold Szechuan flavors.

Preparation time: 15 minutes

Cooking time: 20 minutes

Number of servings: 4

Ingredients:

- 1 large eggplant, cut into bite-sized pieces

- 2 cups broccoli florets

- 2 tablespoons vegetable oil

- 3 cloves garlic, minced

- 1 tablespoon ginger, minced

- 2 tablespoons Szechuan sauce

- 1 tablespoon soy sauce

- 1 tablespoon rice vinegar

- 1 tablespoon honey

- Cooked rice or noodles, for serving

- Sliced green onions and sesame seeds, for garnish (optional)

How to make:

1. Heat vegetable oil in a large skillet or wok over medium-high heat.

2. Add garlic and ginger to the skillet and cook for 1-2 minutes until fragrant.

3. Add eggplant to the skillet and stir-fry for 5-7 minutes until it begins to soften.

4. Add broccoli florets to the skillet and continue to stir-fry for an additional 3-5

minutes until the vegetables are tender but still crisp.

5. In a small bowl, whisk together Szechuan sauce, soy sauce, rice vinegar, and honey.

6. Pour the sauce over the vegetables in the skillet and toss to coat evenly.

7. Cook for an additional 2-3 minutes, stirring constantly, until the sauce has thickened slightly.

8. Serve the stir-fry hot over cooked rice or noodles, garnished with sliced green onions and sesame seeds if desired.

Nutritional info: (per serving)

- Calories: 180

- Fat: 7g

- Carbohydrates: 28g

- Protein: 5g

Thai Basil Vegetable Stir-Fry

Description: A fragrant and vibrant stir-fry featuring an array of vegetables infused with the distinctive flavors of Thai basil and spices.

Preparation time: 15 minutes

Cooking time: 15 minutes

Number of servings: 4

Ingredients:

- 2 cups mixed vegetables (such as bell peppers, snap peas, carrots, and mushrooms), chopped

- 1 cup tofu or chicken, diced (optional)

- 2 tablespoons vegetable oil

- 3 cloves garlic, minced

- 1 tablespoon ginger, minced

- 2 tablespoons Thai basil leaves, chopped

- 2 tablespoons soy sauce

- 1 tablespoon oyster sauce

- 1 tablespoon fish sauce (optional)

- 1 tablespoon brown sugar

- Cooked rice or noodles, for serving

- Sliced red chilies and lime wedges, for garnish (optional)

How to make:

1. Heat vegetable oil in a large skillet or wok over medium-high heat.

2. Add garlic and ginger to the skillet and cook for 1-2 minutes until fragrant.

3. If using tofu or chicken, add it to the skillet and cook until browned on all sides, about 5-7 minutes. Remove from the skillet and set aside.

4. Add mixed vegetables to the skillet and stir-fry for 3-5 minutes until they are tender but still crisp.

5. Return tofu or chicken to the skillet (if using) and add Thai basil leaves.

6. In a small bowl, mix together soy sauce, oyster sauce, fish sauce (if using), and brown sugar.

7. Pour the sauce over the vegetables in the skillet and toss to coat evenly.

8. Cook for an additional 2-3 minutes, stirring constantly, until the sauce has thickened slightly.

9. Serve the stir-fry hot over cooked rice or noodles, garnished with sliced red chilies and lime wedges if desired.

Nutritional info: (per serving)

- Calories: 240

- Fat: 10g

- Carbohydrates: 25g

- Protein: 14g

Spicy Lentil and Sweet Potato Burgers

Description: Bold and flavorful veggie burgers made with hearty lentils and sweet potatoes, kicked up with a spicy twist.

Preparation time: 20 minutes

Cooking time: 30 minutes

Number of servings: 6

Ingredients:

- 1 cup cooked lentils

- 1 cup mashed sweet potatoes

- 1/2 cup breadcrumbs

- 1/4 cup finely chopped onion

- 2 cloves garlic, minced

- 1 teaspoon cumin

- 1 teaspoon paprika

- 1/2 teaspoon chili powder

- Salt and pepper to taste

- 1 tablespoon olive oil

- Burger buns and toppings of choice (lettuce, tomato, avocado, etc.)

How to make:

1. Preheat the oven to 375°F (190°C) and line a baking sheet with parchment paper.

2. In a large mixing bowl, combine cooked lentils, mashed sweet potatoes, breadcrumbs,

onion, garlic, cumin, paprika, chili powder, salt, and pepper. Mix until well combined.

3. Divide the mixture into 6 equal portions and shape each portion into a patty.

4. Heat olive oil in a skillet over medium heat. Cook the patties for 3-4 minutes on each side until golden brown.

5. Transfer the patties to the prepared baking sheet and bake in the preheated oven for 15-20 minutes, until heated through.

6. Serve the burgers on buns with your favorite toppings.

Nutritional info: (per serving)

- Calories: 200

- Fat: 3g

- Carbohydrates: 35g

- Protein: 9g

Black Bean and Quinoa Burgers

Description: Nutritious and satisfying veggie burgers made with black beans and quinoa, packed with protein and fiber.

Preparation time: 20 minutes

Cooking time: 30 minutes

Number of servings: 6

Ingredients:

- 1 cup cooked quinoa

- 1 can (15 oz) black beans, drained and rinsed

- 1/2 cup breadcrumbs

- 1/4 cup finely chopped onion

- 2 cloves garlic, minced

- 1 teaspoon cumin

- 1 teaspoon chili powder

- Salt and pepper to taste

- 1 tablespoon olive oil

- Burger buns and toppings of choice (lettuce, tomato, avocado, etc.)

How to make:

1. In a large mixing bowl, mash the black beans with a fork or potato masher until they are mostly mashed but still have some texture.

2. Add cooked quinoa, breadcrumbs, onion, garlic, cumin, chili powder, salt, and pepper to the bowl. Mix until well combined.

3. Divide the mixture into 6 equal portions and shape each portion into a patty.

4. Heat olive oil in a skillet over medium heat. Cook the patties for 3-4 minutes on each side until golden brown.

5. Serve the burgers on buns with your favorite toppings.

   Nutritional info: (per serving)

- Calories: 220

- Fat: 4g

- Carbohydrates: 36g

- Protein: 10g

Mediterranean Chickpea Burgers

Description: Flavorful veggie burgers inspired by Mediterranean cuisine, featuring chickpeas and aromatic herbs and spices.

Preparation time: 20 minutes

Cooking time: 30 minutes

Number of servings: 6

Ingredients:

- 1 can (15 oz) chickpeas, drained and rinsed

- 1/2 cup breadcrumbs

- 1/4 cup chopped sun-dried tomatoes

- 1/4 cup chopped kalamata olives

- 2 cloves garlic, minced

- 1 tablespoon chopped fresh parsley

- 1 teaspoon dried oregano

- Salt and pepper to taste

- 1 tablespoon olive oil

- Burger buns and toppings of choice (lettuce, tomato, cucumber, tzatziki, etc.)

How to make:

1. In a food processor, pulse chickpeas until coarsely mashed.

2. Transfer mashed chickpeas to a large mixing bowl. Add breadcrumbs, sun-dried tomatoes, olives, garlic, parsley, oregano, salt, and pepper. Mix until well combined.

3. Divide the mixture into 6 equal portions and shape each portion into a patty.

4. Heat olive oil in a skillet over medium heat. Cook the patties for 3-4 minutes on each side until golden brown.

5. Serve the burgers on buns with your favorite toppings.

Nutritional info: (per serving)

- Calories: 210

- Fat: 5g

- Carbohydrates: 32g

- Protein: 9g

Smoky Beet and Walnut Burgers

Description: Vibrant and flavorful veggie burgers made with earthy beets and crunchy walnuts, infused with smoky undertones.

Preparation time: 20 minutes

Cooking time: 30 minutes

Number of servings: 6

Ingredients:

- 2 cups grated beets

- 1 cup cooked brown rice

- 1/2 cup chopped walnuts

- 1/4 cup breadcrumbs

- 1/4 cup chopped fresh cilantro

- 2 cloves garlic, minced

- 1 teaspoon smoked paprika

- 1/2 teaspoon cumin

- Salt and pepper to taste

- 1 tablespoon olive oil

- Burger buns and toppings of choice (lettuce, tomato, avocado, etc.)

How to make:

1. In a large mixing bowl, combine grated beets, cooked brown rice, chopped walnuts, breadcrumbs, cilantro, garlic, smoked paprika, cumin, salt, and pepper. Mix until well combined.

2. Divide the mixture into 6 equal portions and shape each portion into a patty.

3. Heat olive oil in a skillet over medium heat. Cook the patties for 3-4 minutes on each side until golden brown.

4. Serve the burgers on buns with your favorite toppings.

Nutritional info: (per serving)

- Calories: 220

- Fat: 8g

- Carbohydrates: 30g

- Protein: 7g

Mushroom and Lentil Burgers

Description: Hearty and savory veggie burgers made with a combination of mushrooms and lentils, packed with flavor and protein.

Preparation time: 20 minutes

Cooking time: 30 minutes

Number of servings: 6

Ingredients:

- 1 cup cooked lentils

- 1 cup finely chopped mushrooms

- 1/2 cup breadcrumbs

- 1/4 cup finely chopped onion

- 2 cloves garlic, minced

- 1 tablespoon soy sauce

- 1 teaspoon Worcestershire sauce

- 1/2 teaspoon dried thyme

- Salt and pepper to taste

- 1 tablespoon olive oil

- Burger buns and toppings of choice (lettuce, tomato, onion, etc.)

How to make:

1. In a large mixing bowl, combine cooked lentils, chopped mushrooms, breadcrumbs, onion, garlic, soy sauce, Worcestershire sauce, thyme, salt, and pepper. Mix until well combined.

2. Divide the mixture into 6 equal portions and shape each portion into a patty.

3. Heat olive oil in a skillet over medium heat. Cook the patties for 3-4 minutes on each side until golden brown.

4. Serve the burgers on buns with your favorite toppings.

Nutritional info: (per serving)

- Calories: 180

- Fat: 4g

- Carbohydrates: 28g

- Protein: 8g

Buddha Bowl with Roasted Veggies and Tahini Sauce

Description: A nourishing bowl filled with an assortment of roasted vegetables, grains, and a creamy tahini sauce, perfect for a wholesome meal.

Preparation time: 15 minutes

Cooking time: 30 minutes

Number of servings: 4

Ingredients:

- 2 cups mixed vegetables (such as broccoli, cauliflower, carrots, and bell peppers), chopped

- 1 cup cooked quinoa

- 1 cup cooked chickpeas

- 2 tablespoons olive oil

- 1 teaspoon garlic powder

- 1 teaspoon paprika

- Salt and pepper to taste

- 1/4 cup tahini

- 2 tablespoons lemon juice

- 2 tablespoons water

- 1 tablespoon maple syrup or honey (optional)

- Fresh parsley or cilantro, for garnish (optional)

- Sesame seeds, for garnish (optional)

How to make:

1. Preheat the oven to 400°F (200°C) and line a baking sheet with parchment paper.

2. In a large mixing bowl, toss mixed vegetables with olive oil, garlic powder, paprika, salt, and pepper until evenly coated.

3. Spread the vegetables in a single layer on the prepared baking sheet. Roast in the preheated

oven for 20-25 minutes, or until tender and slightly browned.

4. In a small bowl, whisk together tahini, lemon juice, water, and maple syrup or honey (if using) until smooth and creamy. Adjust the consistency with more water if needed.

5. Assemble the Buddha bowls by dividing cooked quinoa, roasted vegetables, and chickpeas among serving bowls.

6. Drizzle tahini sauce over the bowls and garnish with fresh parsley or cilantro and sesame seeds if desired.

7. Serve the Buddha bowls immediately and enjoy!

Nutritional info: (per serving)

- Calories: 320

- Fat: 15g

- Carbohydrates: 40g

- Protein: 12g

Mexican Quinoa Bowl with Black Beans and Avocado

Description: A vibrant and flavorful bowl featuring Mexican-inspired quinoa, black beans, avocado, and fresh toppings, perfect for a satisfying meal.

Preparation time: 15 minutes

Cooking time: 20 minutes

Number of servings: 4

Ingredients:

- 1 cup quinoa, rinsed

- 1 can (15 oz) black beans, drained and rinsed

- 1 cup corn kernels (fresh, canned, or frozen)

- 1 cup cherry tomatoes, halved

- 1 avocado, sliced

- 1/4 cup chopped red onion

- 1/4 cup chopped fresh cilantro

- Juice of 1 lime

- 1 teaspoon chili powder

- 1/2 teaspoon cumin

- Salt and pepper to taste

- Optional toppings: sliced jalapeños, salsa, Greek yogurt or sour cream

How to make:

1. In a medium saucepan, combine quinoa and 2 cups of water. Bring to a boil, then reduce heat to low, cover, and simmer for 15-20 minutes, or until quinoa is cooked and water is absorbed. Remove from heat and fluff with a fork.

2. In a large mixing bowl, combine cooked quinoa, black beans, corn, cherry tomatoes, avocado, red onion, and cilantro.

3. Drizzle lime juice over the mixture and sprinkle with chili powder, cumin, salt, and pepper. Toss until evenly coated.

4. Divide the quinoa mixture among serving bowls.

5. Serve the Mexican quinoa bowls with optional toppings such as sliced jalapeños, salsa, Greek yogurt or sour cream.

Nutritional info: (per serving)

- Calories: 320

- Fat: 10g

- Carbohydrates: 50g

- Protein: 12g

Mediterranean Farro Bowl with Hummus and Vegetables

Description: A hearty and flavorful bowl featuring Mediterranean-inspired farro, creamy hummus, and a variety of fresh vegetables, perfect for a wholesome meal.

Preparation time: 15 minutes

Cooking time: 25 minutes

Number of servings: 4

Ingredients:

- 1 cup farro, rinsed

- 2 cups vegetable broth or water

- 1 cup cherry tomatoes, halved

- 1 cucumber, diced

- 1 bell pepper, diced

- 1/4 cup sliced kalamata olives

- 1/4 cup crumbled feta cheese (optional)

- 1/4 cup chopped fresh parsley

- Juice of 1 lemon

- 2 tablespoons extra virgin olive oil

- Salt and pepper to taste

- 1 cup hummus

- Optional toppings: sliced red onion, chopped fresh mint, toasted pine nuts

How to make:

1. In a medium saucepan, combine farro and vegetable broth or water. Bring to a boil, then reduce heat to low, cover, and simmer for 20-25 minutes, or until farro is tender and water is absorbed. Remove from heat and let cool slightly.

2. In a large mixing bowl, combine cooked farro, cherry tomatoes, cucumber, bell pepper, olives, feta cheese (if using), and parsley.

3. Drizzle lemon juice and olive oil over the mixture. Season with salt and pepper to taste. Toss until evenly coated.

4. Divide the farro mixture among serving bowls.

5. Top each bowl with a generous dollop of hummus.

6. Serve the Mediterranean farro bowls with optional toppings such as sliced red onion, chopped fresh mint, and toasted pine nuts.

Nutritional info: (per serving)

- Calories: 380

- Fat: 16g

- Carbohydrates: 48g

- Protein: 12g

Harvest Bowl with Roasted Sweet Potatoes and Wild Rice

Description: A comforting and nourishing bowl featuring roasted sweet potatoes, hearty wild rice, and a variety of seasonal vegetables, perfect for a cozy meal.

Preparation time: 15 minutes

Cooking time: 30 minutes

Number of servings: 4

Ingredients:

- 2 cups cubed sweet potatoes

- 1 cup wild rice, rinsed

- 2 cups vegetable broth or water

- 2 cups mixed greens (such as spinach, kale, or arugula)

- 1 cup cooked chickpeas

- 1/4 cup dried cranberries

- 1/4 cup chopped pecans or walnuts, toasted

- 2 tablespoons olive oil

- 1 tablespoon maple syrup

- 1 teaspoon cinnamon

- Salt and pepper to taste

- Balsamic glaze or dressing of choice (optional)

How to make:

1. Preheat the oven to 400°F (200°C) and line a baking sheet with parchment paper.

2. In a large mixing bowl, toss cubed sweet potatoes with olive oil, maple syrup, cinnamon, salt, and pepper until evenly coated.

3. Spread the sweet potatoes in a single layer on the prepared baking sheet. Roast in the preheated oven for 25-30 minutes, or until tender and slightly caramelized.

4. In a medium saucepan, combine wild rice and vegetable broth or water. Bring to a boil, then reduce heat to low, cover, and simmer for 35-40 minutes, or until rice is tender and water is absorbed. Remove from heat and let cool slightly.

5. Divide cooked wild rice among serving bowls.

6. Top each bowl with roasted sweet potatoes, mixed greens, cooked chickpeas, dried cranberries, and toasted pecans or walnuts.

7. Drizzle with balsamic glaze or dressing of choice if desired.

8. Serve the harvest bowls warm and enjoy!

Nutritional info: (per serving)

- Calories: 380

- Fat: 12g

- Carbohydrates: 60g

- Protein: 10g

Thai Peanut Nourish Bowl with Crispy Tofu

Description: A vibrant and flavorful bowl featuring crispy tofu, colorful vegetables, and a creamy Thai peanut sauce, perfect for a satisfying and nourishing meal.

Preparation time: 20 minutes

Cooking time: 25 minutes

Number of servings: 4

Ingredients:

- 1 block (14 oz) extra firm tofu, drained and pressed

- 2 cups mixed vegetables (such as bell peppers, broccoli, carrots, and snap peas), chopped

- 1 cup cooked brown rice or quinoa

- 1/4 cup chopped green onions

- 1/4 cup chopped cilantro

- 1/4 cup chopped peanuts

- 2 tablespoons sesame seeds

- 2 tablespoons vegetable oil

- Salt and pepper to taste

  For the Thai Peanut Sauce:

- 1/4 cup peanut butter

- 2 tablespoons soy sauce

- 1 tablespoon maple syrup or honey

- 1 tablespoon rice vinegar

- 1 teaspoon sesame oil

- 1 teaspoon grated ginger

- 1 clove garlic, minced

- Water, as needed to thin

How to make:

1. Preheat the oven to 400°F (200°C). Cut pressed tofu into cubes and place on a parchment-lined baking sheet. Drizzle with 1 tablespoon of vegetable oil and season with salt and pepper. Bake for 25-30 minutes, flipping halfway through, until tofu is crispy and golden brown.

2. In a small bowl, whisk together all the ingredients for the Thai peanut sauce until smooth. Add water as needed to thin the sauce to your desired consistency.

3. In a large skillet or wok, heat the remaining tablespoon of vegetable oil over medium-

high heat. Add mixed vegetables and stir-fry for 3-5 minutes until tender but still crisp.

4. Divide cooked rice or quinoa among serving bowls. Top with crispy tofu, stir-fried vegetables, chopped green onions, cilantro, chopped peanuts, and sesame seeds.

5. Drizzle Thai peanut sauce over the bowls or serve on the side.

6. Serve the Thai peanut nourish bowls immediately and enjoy!

Nutritional info: (per serving)

- Calories: 420

- Fat: 24g

- Carbohydrates: 35g

- Protein: 22g

Vegan Lasagna with Tofu Ricotta

Description: A comforting and hearty vegan lasagna made with layers of marinara sauce, tofu ricotta, and tender lasagna noodles, perfect for a satisfying meal.

Preparation time: 30 minutes

Cooking time: 1 hour

Number of servings: 8

Ingredients:

- 1 box (12 oz) lasagna noodles (preferably whole wheat or gluten-free)

- 2 cups marinara sauce

- 1 block (14 oz) firm tofu, drained

- 2 tablespoons nutritional yeast

- 1 tablespoon lemon juice

- 1 teaspoon dried basil

- 1 teaspoon dried oregano

- 1/2 teaspoon garlic powder

- Salt and pepper to taste

- 2 cups fresh spinach leaves

- 1 cup sliced mushrooms

- 1 cup diced bell peppers

- 1 cup shredded vegan cheese (optional)

How to make:

1. Preheat the oven to 375°F (190°C). Cook lasagna noodles according to package instructions, then drain and set aside.

2. In a food processor, combine drained tofu, nutritional yeast, lemon juice, dried basil, dried oregano, garlic powder, salt, and pepper. Blend until smooth and creamy to make the tofu ricotta.

3. In a baking dish, spread a thin layer of marinara sauce on the bottom. Arrange a layer of cooked lasagna noodles on top.

4. Spread half of the tofu ricotta over the noodles, then layer with fresh spinach leaves, sliced mushrooms, and diced bell peppers.

5. Repeat the layers with marinara sauce, lasagna noodles, remaining tofu ricotta, and vegetables.

6. Top the lasagna with a final layer of marinara sauce and sprinkle with shredded vegan cheese if using.

7. Cover the baking dish with foil and bake in the preheated oven for 30 minutes.

8. Remove the foil and bake for an additional 15-20 minutes, or until the lasagna is hot and bubbly.

9. Let the lasagna cool for a few minutes before slicing and serving.

Nutritional info: (per serving)

- Calories: 320

- Fat: 8g

- Carbohydrates: 45g

- Protein: 18g

Vegetable Pasta Primavera

Description: A light and flavorful pasta dish featuring a medley of seasonal vegetables tossed in a garlic-infused olive oil sauce, perfect for a quick and easy meal.

Preparation time: 20 minutes

Cooking time: 15 minutes

Number of servings: 4

Ingredients:

- 8 oz pasta of choice (such as spaghetti, fettuccine, or penne)
- 2 tablespoons olive oil

- 3 cloves garlic, minced

- 2 cups mixed vegetables (such as cherry tomatoes, zucchini, bell peppers, and asparagus), chopped

- 1/4 cup chopped fresh basil

- 1/4 cup chopped fresh parsley

- Juice of 1 lemon

- Salt and pepper to taste

- Grated vegan Parmesan cheese (optional)

How to make:

1. Cook pasta according to package instructions until al dente. Drain and set aside.

2. In a large skillet, heat olive oil over medium heat. Add minced garlic and cook for 1-2 minutes until fragrant.

3. Add mixed vegetables to the skillet and sauté for 5-7 minutes until tender but still crisp.

4. Stir in cooked pasta, chopped basil, chopped parsley, and lemon juice. Toss until well combined.

5. Season with salt and pepper to taste.

6. Serve the vegetable pasta primavera hot, garnished with grated vegan Parmesan cheese if desired.

Nutritional info: (per serving)

- Calories: 280

- Fat: 8g

- Carbohydrates: 45g

- Protein: 8g

Lentil Bolognese over Zucchini Noodles

Description: A nutritious and flavorful twist on classic Bolognese sauce, featuring hearty lentils served over spiralized zucchini noodles, perfect for a light and satisfying meal.

Preparation time: 15 minutes

Cooking time: 30 minutes

Number of servings: 4

Ingredients:

- 2 medium zucchini

- 1 cup dried green or brown lentils

- 2 cups vegetable broth or water

- 2 tablespoons olive oil

- 1 onion, diced

- 2 cloves garlic, minced

- 1 carrot, diced

- 1 stalk celery, diced

- 1 can (14 oz) crushed tomatoes

- 1 teaspoon dried oregano

- 1 teaspoon dried basil

- Salt and pepper to taste

- Chopped fresh parsley for garnish (optional)

How to make:

1. Use a spiralizer to spiralize the zucchini into noodles. Set aside.

2. Rinse lentils under cold water and drain. In a medium saucepan, combine lentils and vegetable broth or water. Bring to a boil, then

reduce heat to low, cover, and simmer for 20-25 minutes, or until lentils are tender.

3. In a large skillet, heat olive oil over medium heat. Add diced onion, minced garlic, diced carrot, and diced celery. Sauté for 5-7 minutes until vegetables are softened.

4. Stir in crushed tomatoes, dried oregano, dried basil, salt, and pepper. Simmer for 10-15 minutes, stirring occasionally.

5. Once lentils are cooked, add them to the skillet with the tomato sauce. Stir to combine and simmer for an additional 5-10 minutes.

6. In a separate skillet, heat a little olive oil over medium heat. Add spiralized zucchini noodles and sauté for 2-3 minutes until just tender.

7. Serve the lentil Bolognese over the sautéed zucchini noodles.

8. Garnish with chopped fresh parsley if desired.

Nutritional info: (per serving)

- Calories: 280

- Fat: 6g

- Carbohydrates: 45g

- Protein: 15g

Baked Vegan Mac and Cheese

Description: A creamy and comforting vegan version of classic macaroni and cheese, baked to perfection with a crunchy breadcrumb topping.

Preparation time: 20 minutes

Cooking time: 25 minutes

Number of servings: 6

Ingredients:

- 8 oz elbow macaroni or pasta of choice

- 2 cups unsweetened almond milk (or any non-dairy milk)

- 1/4 cup nutritional yeast

- 1/4 cup all-purpose flour (or gluten-free flour)

- 2 tablespoons vegan butter or olive oil

- 1 teaspoon garlic powder

- 1 teaspoon onion powder

- 1/2 teaspoon mustard powder

- Salt and pepper to taste

- 1 cup shredded vegan cheese

- 1/2 cup breadcrumbs

- Fresh parsley for garnish (optional)

How to make:

1. Preheat the oven to 375°F (190°C) and lightly grease a baking dish.

2. Cook macaroni according to package instructions until al dente. Drain and set aside.

3. In a saucepan, melt vegan butter over medium heat. Whisk in flour to form a roux, then gradually whisk in almond milk until smooth.

4. Stir in nutritional yeast, garlic powder, onion
    powder, mustard powder, salt, and pepper.
    Cook for 5-7 minutes, stirring constantly,
    until the sauce thickens.

5. Remove the saucepan from heat and stir in
    shredded vegan cheese until melted and
    smooth.

6. In a large mixing bowl, combine cooked
    macaroni with the cheese sauce until evenly
    coated.

7. Transfer the mac and cheese mixture to the
    prepared baking dish.

8. In a small bowl, combine breadcrumbs with
    a little olive oil or melted vegan butter.
    Sprinkle the breadcrumb mixture evenly over
    the top of the mac and cheese.

9. Bake in the preheated oven for 20-25 minutes, or until the top is golden brown and the sauce is bubbly.

10. Garnish with fresh parsley if desired before serving.

Nutritional info: (per serving)

- Calories: 320

- Fat: 10g

- Carbohydrates: 45g

- Protein: 12g

Vegetable Stuffed Shells with Cashew Cream Sauce

Description: Creamy and indulgent stuffed pasta shells filled with a savory vegetable mixture and topped with a rich cashew cream sauce, perfect for a special occasion or a cozy dinner.

Preparation time: 30 minutes

Cooking time: 30 minutes

Number of servings: 6

Ingredients:

- 18 jumbo pasta shells

- 2 cups mixed vegetables (such as spinach, mushrooms, bell peppers, and zucchini), chopped

- 1 cup raw cashews, soaked in hot water for 1 hour

- 1 cup vegetable broth

- 2 cloves garlic, minced

- 1/4 cup nutritional yeast

- 2 tablespoons lemon juice

- 1 teaspoon onion powder

- 1/2 teaspoon dried basil

- Salt and pepper to taste

- Fresh parsley for garnish (optional)

How to make:

1. Cook pasta shells according to package instructions until al dente. Drain and set aside.

2. In a large skillet, sauté mixed vegetables and minced garlic over medium heat for 5-7 minutes until tender. Remove from heat and let cool slightly.

3. In a blender, combine soaked cashews, vegetable broth, nutritional yeast, lemon juice, onion powder, dried basil, salt, and pepper. Blend until smooth and creamy to make the cashew cream sauce.

4. Preheat the oven to 375°F (190°C) and lightly grease a baking dish.

5. Stuff cooked pasta shells with the sautéed vegetable mixture and arrange them in the prepared baking dish.

6. Pour cashew cream sauce over the stuffed shells, covering them evenly.

7. Cover the baking dish with foil and bake in the preheated oven for 20-25 minutes, or until the sauce is bubbly and heated through.

8. Garnish with fresh parsley if desired before serving.

Nutritional info: (per serving)

- Calories: 350

- Fat: 18g

- Carbohydrates: 35g

- Protein: 14g

Roasted Vegetable Pasta Bake

Description: A comforting and flavorful pasta bake featuring roasted vegetables, marinara sauce, and melted cheese, baked to perfection for a satisfying meal.

Preparation time: 20 minutes

Cooking time: 40 minutes

Number of servings: 6

Ingredients:

- 8 oz penne pasta or pasta of choice

- 2 cups mixed vegetables (such as bell peppers, zucchini, cherry tomatoes, and red onion), chopped

- 2 cups marinara sauce

- 1 cup shredded mozzarella cheese (or vegan cheese)

- 1/4 cup grated Parmesan cheese (or vegan Parmesan)

- 2 tablespoons olive oil

- 2 cloves garlic, minced

- 1 teaspoon dried oregano

- 1 teaspoon dried basil

- Salt and pepper to taste

- Fresh basil leaves for garnish (optional)

How to make:

1. Preheat the oven to 375°F (190°C) and lightly grease a baking dish.

2. Cook pasta according to package instructions until al dente. Drain and set aside.

3. In a large mixing bowl, toss chopped vegetables with olive oil, minced garlic, dried oregano, dried basil, salt, and pepper until evenly coated.

4. Spread the seasoned vegetables in a single layer on a baking sheet. Roast in the

preheated oven for 20-25 minutes, or until tender and slightly caramelized.

5. In a large mixing bowl, combine cooked pasta, roasted vegetables, and marinara sauce. Toss until well combined.

6. Transfer the pasta mixture to the prepared baking dish.

7. Sprinkle shredded mozzarella cheese and grated Parmesan cheese over the top.

8. Bake in the preheated oven for 20-25 minutes, or until the cheese is melted and bubbly.

9. Garnish with fresh basil leaves if desired before serving.

Nutritional info: (per serving)

- Calories: 320

- Fat: 10g

- Carbohydrates: 45g

- Protein: 12g

Butternut Squash Alfredo with Spinach

Description: A creamy and velvety Alfredo sauce made with roasted butternut squash and spinach, tossed with fettuccine pasta for a luxurious and comforting meal.

Preparation time: 20 minutes

Cooking time: 40 minutes

Number of servings: 4

Ingredients:

- 8 oz fettuccine pasta

- 2 cups diced butternut squash

- 2 cups fresh spinach leaves

- 1 cup unsweetened almond milk (or any non-dairy milk)

- 1/2 cup raw cashews, soaked in hot water for 1 hour

- 2 cloves garlic, minced

- 2 tablespoons nutritional yeast

- 1 tablespoon lemon juice

- 1/2 teaspoon onion powder

- Salt and pepper to taste

- Pinch of nutmeg (optional)

- Fresh parsley for garnish (optional)

How to make:

1. Preheat the oven to 400°F (200°C) and line a baking sheet with parchment paper.

2. Arrange diced butternut squash on the prepared baking sheet in a single layer. Roast in the preheated oven for 20-25 minutes, or until tender and caramelized.

3. Cook fettuccine pasta according to package instructions until al dente. Drain and set aside.

4. In a blender, combine roasted butternut squash, soaked cashews, almond milk, minced garlic, nutritional yeast, lemon juice, onion powder, salt, pepper, and nutmeg (if using). Blend until smooth and creamy to make the Alfredo sauce.

5. In a large skillet, heat the Alfredo sauce over medium heat. Add fresh spinach leaves and cooked fettuccine pasta. Toss until the pasta is evenly coated and the spinach is wilted.

6. Serve the butternut squash Alfredo hot, garnished with fresh parsley if desired.

   Nutritional info: (per serving)

- Calories: 380

- Fat: 12g

- Carbohydrates: 55g

- Protein: 15g

Mexican Lentil and Sweet Potato Casserole

Description: A hearty and flavorful casserole featuring layers of Mexican-spiced lentils, sweet potatoes, corn, and melted cheese, baked to perfection for a comforting meal.

Preparation time: 30 minutes

Cooking time: 45 minutes

Number of servings: 6

Ingredients:

- 1 cup dry brown or green lentils
- 2 cups vegetable broth or water
- 2 cups diced sweet potatoes
- 1 cup corn kernels (fresh, canned, or frozen)
- 1 can (15 oz) black beans, drained and rinsed

- 1 cup salsa

- 1 teaspoon chili powder

- 1/2 teaspoon cumin

- 1/2 teaspoon paprika

- Salt and pepper to taste

- 1 cup shredded cheddar cheese (or vegan cheese)

- Fresh cilantro for garnish (optional)

- Sliced avocado for serving (optional)

How to make:

1. In a medium saucepan, combine dry lentils and vegetable broth or water. Bring to a boil, then reduce heat to low, cover, and simmer for 20-25 minutes, or until lentils are tender.

2. Preheat the oven to 375°F (190°C) and lightly grease a baking dish.

3. In a large mixing bowl, combine cooked lentils, diced sweet potatoes, corn kernels, black beans, salsa, chili powder, cumin, paprika, salt, and pepper. Stir until well combined.

4. Transfer the lentil and sweet potato mixture to the prepared baking dish. Spread it out into an even layer.

5. Sprinkle shredded cheddar cheese over the top.

6. Cover the baking dish with foil and bake in the preheated oven for 30 minutes.

7. Remove the foil and bake for an additional 10-15 minutes, or until the cheese is melted and bubbly.

8. Garnish with fresh cilantro and serve with sliced avocado if desired.

Nutritional info: (per serving)

- Calories: 320

- Fat: 8g

- Carbohydrates: 50g

- Protein: 15g

Eggplant Rollatini with Cashew Ricotta

Description: Elegant and delicious eggplant rollatini filled with creamy cashew ricotta cheese and baked in marinara sauce, perfect for a special dinner or a festive occasion.

Preparation time: 30 minutes

Cooking time: 45 minutes

Number of servings: 4

Ingredients:

- 1 large eggplant, thinly sliced lengthwise

- 2 cups marinara sauce

- 1 cup raw cashews, soaked in hot water for 1 hour

- 1/4 cup nutritional yeast

- 2 tablespoons lemon juice

- 1 clove garlic, minced

- 1 tablespoon chopped fresh basil

- 1 tablespoon chopped fresh parsley

- Salt and pepper to taste

- Olive oil for brushing

- Vegan Parmesan cheese for garnish (optional)

How to make:

1. Preheat the oven to 375°F (190°C) and lightly grease a baking dish.

2. Lay eggplant slices on a baking sheet and brush both sides with olive oil. Bake in the preheated oven for 15-20 minutes, or until tender and slightly golden brown. Remove from oven and let cool slightly.

3. In a blender, combine soaked cashews, nutritional yeast, lemon juice, minced garlic,

chopped basil, chopped parsley, salt, and pepper. Blend until smooth and creamy to make the cashew ricotta cheese.

4. Spread a thin layer of marinara sauce on the bottom of the prepared baking dish.

5. Place a spoonful of cashew ricotta cheese on one end of each eggplant slice and roll it up. Place the rolled eggplant seam side down in the baking dish.

6. Pour the remaining marinara sauce over the eggplant rollatini, covering them evenly.

7. Cover the baking dish with foil and bake in the preheated oven for 25-30 minutes, or until the sauce is bubbly.

8. Garnish with vegan Parmesan cheese if desired before serving.

Nutritional info: (per serving)

- Calories: 280

- Fat: 16g

- Carbohydrates: 25g

- Protein: 10g

Vegan Shepherd's Pie with Lentils and Mushrooms

Description: A hearty and comforting vegan version of classic shepherd's pie, featuring a savory filling of lentils, mushrooms, and vegetables topped with creamy mashed potatoes.

Preparation time: 30 minutes

Cooking time: 40 minutes

Number of servings: 6

Ingredients:

- 4 large potatoes, peeled and diced

- 1 tablespoon olive oil

- 1 onion, diced

- 2 cloves garlic, minced

- 2 carrots, diced

- 2 celery stalks, diced

- 8 oz mushrooms, chopped

- 1 cup cooked green or brown lentils

- 1 cup vegetable broth

- 1 tablespoon tomato paste

- 1 teaspoon dried thyme

- 1 teaspoon dried rosemary

- Salt and pepper to taste

- Fresh parsley for garnish (optional)

How to make:

1. Place diced potatoes in a large pot of water. Bring to a boil and cook until potatoes are fork-tender, about 15-20 minutes. Drain and set aside.

2. Preheat the oven to 375°F (190°C) and lightly grease a baking dish.

3. In a large skillet, heat olive oil over medium heat. Add diced onion and minced garlic, and sauté until softened, about 3-4 minutes.

4. Add diced carrots, diced celery, and chopped mushrooms to the skillet. Sauté for another 5-7 minutes until vegetables are tender.

5. Stir in cooked lentils, vegetable broth, tomato paste, dried thyme, dried rosemary, salt, and pepper. Simmer for 5-7 minutes until the mixture thickens slightly.

6. Transfer the lentil and mushroom mixture to the prepared baking dish and spread it out into an even layer.

7. In a mixing bowl, mash cooked potatoes until smooth. Season with salt and pepper to taste.

8. Spread mashed potatoes over the lentil and mushroom mixture in the baking dish, covering it completely.

9. Bake in the preheated oven for 20-25 minutes, or until the top is golden brown and the filling is bubbly.

10. Garnish with fresh parsley before serving.

Nutritional info: (per serving)

- Calories: 280

- Fat: 6g

- Carbohydrates: 45g

- Protein: 12g

Chapter 5

Sides and Small Bites

Roasted Brussels Sprouts with Balsamic Glaze

Description: Tender roasted Brussels sprouts drizzled with a sweet and tangy balsamic glaze, perfect as a flavorful side dish.

Preparation time: 10 minutes

Cooking time: 25 minutes

Number of servings: 4

Ingredients:

- 1 lb Brussels sprouts, trimmed and halved

- 2 tablespoons olive oil

- Salt and pepper to taste

- 2 tablespoons balsamic vinegar

- 1 tablespoon honey or maple syrup (for vegan option)

- 1 teaspoon Dijon mustard (optional)

How to make:

1. Preheat your oven to 400°F (200°C).

2. In a large bowl, toss the Brussels sprouts with olive oil, salt, and pepper until evenly coated.

3. Spread the Brussels sprouts in a single layer on a baking sheet.

4. Roast in the preheated oven for about 20-25 minutes or until they are tender and slightly caramelized.

5. In a small saucepan, combine the balsamic vinegar, honey or maple syrup, and Dijon mustard. Simmer over medium heat until the glaze thickens slightly, about 5 minutes.

6. Drizzle the balsamic glaze over the roasted Brussels sprouts before serving.

Nutritional info: (per serving)

- Calories: 120

- Fat: 7g

- Carbohydrates: 14g

- Fiber: 4g

- Protein: 3g

Sautéed Garlic Green Beans

Description: Crisp green beans tossed in garlic-infused olive oil for a simple and flavorful side dish.

Preparation time: 10 minutes

Cooking time: 10 minutes

Number of servings: 4

Ingredients:

- 1 lb green beans, trimmed

- 2 tablespoons olive oil

- 3 cloves garlic, minced

- Salt and pepper to taste

- Lemon wedges for serving (optional)

How to make:

1. Heat olive oil in a large skillet over medium heat. Add the minced garlic and sauté for 1 minute until fragrant.

2. Add the green beans to the skillet and toss to coat them evenly with the garlic oil.

3. Cook the green beans for about 5-7 minutes, stirring occasionally, until they are tender but still crisp.

4. Season with salt and pepper to taste.

5. Serve the sautéed garlic green beans hot, with lemon wedges if desired.

Nutritional info: (per serving)

- Calories: 80

- Fat: 5g

- Carbohydrates: 8g

- Fiber: 4g

- Protein: 2g

Roasted Root Vegetable Medley

Description: A colorful mix of roasted root vegetables seasoned with herbs, olive oil, and balsamic vinegar.

Preparation time: 15 minutes

Cooking time: 40 minutes

Number of servings: 6

Ingredients:

- 2 carrots, peeled and cut into chunks

- 2 parsnips, peeled and cut into chunks

- 2 beets, peeled and cut into chunks

- 1 sweet potato, peeled and cut into chunks

- 1 red onion, cut into wedges

- 3 tablespoons olive oil

- 2 tablespoons balsamic vinegar

- 2 cloves garlic, minced

- 1 teaspoon dried thyme

- Salt and pepper to taste

- Fresh parsley for garnish (optional)

How to make:

1. Preheat your oven to 400°F (200°C).

2. In a large bowl, toss together the carrots, parsnips, beets, sweet potato, and red onion

with olive oil, balsamic vinegar, minced garlic, dried thyme, salt, and pepper until evenly coated.

3. Spread the vegetable mixture in a single layer on a baking sheet.

4. Roast in the preheated oven for about 35-40 minutes, stirring halfway through, until the vegetables are tender and caramelized.

5. Garnish with fresh parsley before serving, if desired.

Nutritional info: (per serving)

- Calories: 150

- Fat: 7g

- Carbohydrates: 21g

- Fiber: 5g

- Protein: 2g

Baked Sweet Potato Fries

Description: Crispy sweet potato fries seasoned with spices and baked to perfection, a healthier alternative to traditional fries.

Preparation time: 10 minutes

Cooking time: 25 minutes

Number of servings: 4

Ingredients:

- 2 large sweet potatoes, peeled and cut into fries

- 2 tablespoons olive oil

- 1 teaspoon paprika

- 1/2 teaspoon garlic powder

- 1/2 teaspoon onion powder

- Salt and pepper to taste

- Fresh parsley for garnish (optional)

How to make:

1. Preheat your oven to 425°F (220°C).

2. In a large bowl, toss the sweet potato fries with olive oil, paprika, garlic powder, onion powder, salt, and pepper until evenly coated.

3. Spread the sweet potato fries in a single layer on a baking sheet lined with parchment paper.

4. Bake in the preheated oven for about 20-25 minutes, flipping halfway through, until the fries are crispy and golden brown.

5. Garnish with fresh parsley before serving, if desired.

Nutritional info: (per serving)

- Calories: 150

- Fat: 7g

- Carbohydrates: 21g

- Fiber: 4g

- Protein: 2g

Vegan Potato Salad

Description: Creamy and flavorful potato salad made with a dairy-free dressing and plenty of fresh herbs and vegetables.

Preparation time: 15 minutes

Cooking time: 20 minutes

Number of servings: 6

Ingredients:

- 2 lbs potatoes, peeled and diced

- 1/2 cup vegan mayonnaise

- 2 tablespoons Dijon mustard

- 1 tablespoon apple cider vinegar

- 1/4 cup chopped fresh dill

- 1/4 cup chopped fresh parsley

- 2 celery stalks, finely chopped

- 1/2 red onion, finely chopped

- Salt and pepper to taste

- Paprika for garnish (optional)

How to make:

1. Place the diced potatoes in a large pot of salted water. Bring to a boil and cook for about 15-20 minutes, or until the potatoes are fork-tender.

2. Drain the potatoes and let them cool slightly.

3. In a large bowl, whisk together the vegan mayonnaise, Dijon mustard, apple cider vinegar, chopped dill, chopped parsley, chopped celery, and chopped red onion.

4. Add the cooked potatoes to the bowl and toss until they are evenly coated with the dressing.

5. Season with salt and pepper to taste.

6. Refrigerate the potato salad for at least 1 hour before serving to allow the flavors to meld.

7. Sprinkle with paprika before serving, if desired.

Nutritional info: (per serving)

- Calories: 200

- Fat: 6g

- Carbohydrates: 32g

- Fiber: 4g

- Protein: 4g

Loaded Baked Potato Wedges

Description: Crispy potato wedges topped with melted cheese, crispy bacon, sour cream, and green onions, a delicious twist on classic loaded baked potatoes.

Preparation time: 15 minutes

Cooking time: 30 minutes

Number of servings: 4

Ingredients:

- 2 large russet potatoes, scrubbed and cut into wedges

- 2 tablespoons olive oil

- Salt and pepper to taste

- 1 cup shredded cheddar cheese

- 4 slices cooked bacon, crumbled

- 1/4 cup sour cream

- 2 green onions, thinly sliced

- Chopped fresh parsley for garnish (optional)

How to make:

1. Preheat your oven to 425°F (220°C).

2. In a large bowl, toss the potato wedges with olive oil, salt, and pepper until evenly coated.

3. Spread the potato wedges in a single layer on a baking sheet lined with parchment paper.

4. Bake in the preheated oven for about 25-30 minutes, flipping halfway through, until the wedges are golden brown and crispy.

5. Remove the potato wedges from the oven and sprinkle them with shredded cheddar cheese. Return to the oven and bake for an additional 2-3 minutes, or until the cheese is melted and bubbly.

6. Remove from the oven and top the loaded
   potato wedges with crumbled bacon, sour
   cream, sliced green onions, and chopped
   fresh parsley, if desired.

Nutritional info: (per serving)

- Calories: 300

- Fat: 18g

- Carbohydrates: 20g

- Fiber: 2g

- Protein: 14g

Muhammara (Roasted Red Pepper and Walnut Dip)

Description: A vibrant and flavorful dip made with roasted red peppers, toasted walnuts, and aromatic spices, perfect for dipping pita bread or veggies.

Preparation time: 15 minutes

Cooking time: 10 minutes

Number of servings: 6

Ingredients:

- 2 large red bell peppers
- 1 cup walnuts, toasted
- 2 cloves garlic, minced
- 2 tablespoons lemon juice
- 2 tablespoons olive oil
- 1 tablespoon pomegranate molasses (or honey)
- 1 teaspoon ground cumin

- 1/2 teaspoon smoked paprika

- Salt and pepper to taste

- Chopped fresh parsley for garnish (optional)

How to make:

1. Preheat your broiler to high. Place the red bell peppers on a baking sheet and broil, turning occasionally, until the skins are charred and blistered, about 8-10 minutes.

2. Transfer the roasted red peppers to a bowl and cover with plastic wrap. Let them steam for 5 minutes, then peel off the charred skins and remove the seeds and stems.

3. In a food processor, combine the roasted red peppers, toasted walnuts, minced garlic, lemon juice, olive oil, pomegranate molasses,

ground cumin, smoked paprika, salt, and pepper. Blend until smooth.

4. Transfer the muhammara to a serving bowl and garnish with chopped fresh parsley, if desired.

5. Serve the muhammara with pita bread, crackers, or fresh vegetables for dipping.

Nutritional info: (per serving)

- Calories: 180

- Fat: 15g

- Carbohydrates: 9g

- Fiber: 2g

- Protein: 4g

Cashew Cream Sauce

Description: A creamy and versatile sauce made from cashews, perfect as a dairy-free alternative for pasta, salads, or as a dip.

Preparation time: 5 minutes (plus soaking time)

Cooking time: 5 minutes

Number of servings: 8

Ingredients:

- 1 cup raw cashews, soaked in water for at least 4 hours or overnight

- 1/2 cup water (more as needed)

- 2 tablespoons nutritional yeast

- 1 tablespoon lemon juice

- 1 clove garlic, minced

- Salt and pepper to taste

- Fresh herbs for garnish (optional)

How to make:

1. Drain and rinse the soaked cashews.

2. In a blender, combine the soaked cashews, water, nutritional yeast, lemon juice, minced garlic, salt, and pepper. Blend until smooth and creamy, adding more water as needed to reach your desired consistency.

3. Adjust seasoning to taste with salt and pepper.

4. Transfer the cashew cream sauce to a saucepan and warm over low heat, stirring occasionally, until heated through.

5. Serve the cashew cream sauce drizzled over pasta, salads, or use it as a dip for vegetables.

6. Garnish with fresh herbs, if desired.

Nutritional info: (per serving)

- Calories: 90

- Fat: 7g

- Carbohydrates: 5g

- Fiber: 1g

- Protein: 4g

White Bean and Basil Spread

Description: A creamy and flavorful spread made with white beans, fresh basil, garlic, and lemon juice, perfect for spreading on toast or crackers.

Preparation time: 10 minutes

Cooking time: 0 minutes

Number of servings: 6

Ingredients:

- 1 can (15 oz) white beans, drained and rinsed

- 1/4 cup fresh basil leaves

- 2 cloves garlic, minced

- 2 tablespoons lemon juice

- 2 tablespoons olive oil

- Salt and pepper to taste

- Red pepper flakes for garnish (optional)

How to make:

1. In a food processor, combine the white beans, fresh basil leaves, minced garlic, lemon juice,

olive oil, salt, and pepper. Blend until smooth and creamy.

2. Taste and adjust seasoning as needed with salt, pepper, and additional lemon juice.

3. Transfer the white bean and basil spread to a serving bowl.

4. Garnish with a drizzle of olive oil and a sprinkle of red pepper flakes, if desired.

5. Serve the spread with toast, crackers, or fresh vegetables.

Nutritional info: (per serving)

- Calories: 100

- Fat: 4g

- Carbohydrates: 12g

- Fiber: 3g

- Protein: 4g

Baked Vegetable Spring Rolls with Peanut Dipping Sauce

Description: Crispy baked spring rolls filled with a colorful mix of vegetables, served with a creamy peanut dipping sauce.

Preparation time: 30 minutes

Cooking time: 20 minutes

Number of servings: 4

Ingredients:

For the spring rolls:

- 8 spring roll wrappers

- 2 cups shredded cabbage

- 1 carrot, julienned

- 1 bell pepper, thinly sliced

- 1/2 cup bean sprouts

- 2 green onions, thinly sliced

- 1 tablespoon soy sauce

- 1 tablespoon sesame oil

- 1 teaspoon grated ginger

- 1 clove garlic, minced

- Salt and pepper to taste

- Cooking spray

For the peanut dipping sauce:

- 1/4 cup creamy peanut butter

- 2 tablespoons soy sauce

- 1 tablespoon rice vinegar

- 1 tablespoon maple syrup or honey

- 1 teaspoon sesame oil

- 1 clove garlic, minced

- Water as needed for thinning

How to make:

1. Preheat your oven to 425°F (220°C).

2. In a large bowl, combine the shredded cabbage, julienned carrot, sliced bell pepper, bean sprouts, and sliced green onions.

3. In a small bowl, whisk together the soy sauce, sesame oil, grated ginger, minced garlic, salt, and pepper. Pour the sauce over the vegetable mixture and toss until evenly coated.

4. Place a spring roll wrapper on a clean surface. Spoon about 1/4 cup of the vegetable filling onto the bottom third of the wrapper.

5. Fold the bottom of the wrapper over the filling, then fold in the sides, and roll it up tightly.

6. Place the spring roll seam-side down on a baking sheet lined with parchment paper. Repeat with the remaining wrappers and filling.

7. Lightly spray the spring rolls with cooking spray.

8. Bake in the preheated oven for about 18-20 minutes, or until the spring rolls are golden brown and crispy.

9. While the spring rolls are baking, make the peanut dipping sauce. In a small bowl, whisk together the peanut butter, soy sauce, rice vinegar, maple syrup or honey, sesame oil, minced garlic, and enough water to reach your desired consistency.

10. Serve the baked vegetable spring rolls hot, with the peanut dipping sauce on the side.

    Nutritional info: (per serving, including dipping sauce)

- Calories: 250

- Fat: 10g

- Carbohydrates: 32g

- Fiber: 4g

- Protein: 9g

Chapter 6

Sweet Treats

Vegan Chocolate Cake

Description: Rich and moist chocolate cake made without eggs or dairy, topped with a decadent chocolate ganache.

Preparation time: 15 minutes

Baking time: 30 minutes

Number of servings: 8

Ingredients:

For the cake:

- 1 1/2 cups all-purpose flour

- 1 cup granulated sugar

- 1/4 cup cocoa powder

- 1 teaspoon baking soda

- 1/2 teaspoon salt

- 1 cup brewed coffee, cooled

- 1/3 cup vegetable oil

- 1 tablespoon white or apple cider vinegar

- 1 teaspoon vanilla extract

For the chocolate ganache:

- 1/2 cup dairy-free chocolate chips

- 1/4 cup full-fat coconut milk

How to make:

1. Preheat your oven to 350°F (175°C). Grease

   and flour an 8-inch round cake pan.

2. In a large mixing bowl, whisk together the flour, sugar, cocoa powder, baking soda, and salt.

3. Add the brewed coffee, vegetable oil, vinegar, and vanilla extract to the dry ingredients. Mix until well combined and smooth.

4. Pour the batter into the prepared cake pan and smooth the top with a spatula.

5. Bake in the preheated oven for 25-30 minutes, or until a toothpick inserted into the center comes out clean.

6. Allow the cake to cool in the pan for 10 minutes, then transfer it to a wire rack to cool completely.

For the chocolate ganache:

1. In a small saucepan, heat the coconut milk until it just begins to simmer.

2. Place the chocolate chips in a heatproof bowl and pour the hot coconut milk over them.

3. Let it sit for 2-3 minutes, then whisk until smooth and glossy.

4. Let the ganache cool for a few minutes, then pour it over the cooled cake.

5. Allow the ganache to set before slicing and serving.

Nutritional info: (per serving)

- Calories: 320

- Fat: 15g

- Carbohydrates: 45g

- Fiber: 2g

- Protein: 3g

Oatmeal Raisin Cookies

Description: Chewy and comforting oatmeal cookies studded with sweet raisins and warm spices.

Preparation time: 15 minutes

Baking time: 10-12 minutes per batch

Number of servings: 24 cookies

Ingredients:

- 1 cup rolled oats

- 3/4 cup all-purpose flour

- 1/2 teaspoon baking soda

- 1/2 teaspoon ground cinnamon

- 1/4 teaspoon salt

- 1/2 cup vegan butter, softened

- 1/2 cup brown sugar, packed

- 1/4 cup granulated sugar

- 1 flax egg (1 tablespoon ground flaxseed + 3 tablespoons water)

- 1 teaspoon vanilla extract

- 3/4 cup raisins

How to make:

1. Preheat your oven to 350°F (175°C). Line a baking sheet with parchment paper.

2. In a medium bowl, whisk together the rolled oats, flour, baking soda, cinnamon, and salt.

3. In a large mixing bowl, beat the softened vegan butter, brown sugar, and granulated sugar until creamy.

4. Add the flax egg and vanilla extract to the butter mixture and beat until well combined.

5. Gradually add the dry ingredients to the wet ingredients and mix until just combined.

6. Fold in the raisins until evenly distributed throughout the dough.

7. Drop tablespoonfuls of dough onto the prepared baking sheet, spacing them about 2 inches apart.

8. Bake in the preheated oven for 10-12 minutes, or until the edges are golden brown.

9. Allow the cookies to cool on the baking sheet for 5 minutes before transferring them to a wire rack to cool completely.

Nutritional info: (per cookie)

- Calories: 100

- Fat: 4g

- Carbohydrates: 15g

- Fiber: 1g

- Protein: 1g

Fudgy Brownies

Description: Indulgent and gooey chocolate brownies that are rich in flavor and completely vegan.

Preparation time: 15 minutes

Baking time: 25-30 minutes

Number of servings: 12 brownies

Ingredients:

- 1/2 cup vegan butter, melted

- 1 cup granulated sugar

- 1/2 cup unsweetened applesauce

- 1 teaspoon vanilla extract

- 3/4 cup all-purpose flour

- 1/2 cup cocoa powder

- 1/4 teaspoon salt

- 1/4 teaspoon baking powder

- 1/2 cup dairy-free chocolate chips

How to make:

1. Preheat your oven to 350°F (175°C). Grease and flour an 8-inch square baking pan.

2. In a large mixing bowl, whisk together the melted vegan butter, granulated sugar, applesauce, and vanilla extract until smooth.

3. In a separate bowl, sift together the flour, cocoa powder, salt, and baking powder.

4. Gradually add the dry ingredients to the wet ingredients, mixing until just combined.

5. Fold in the dairy-free chocolate chips until evenly distributed throughout the batter.

6. Pour the batter into the prepared baking pan and spread it out evenly with a spatula.

7. Bake in the preheated oven for 25-30 minutes, or until a toothpick inserted into the center comes out with a few moist crumbs.

8. Allow the brownies to cool completely in the
    pan before slicing and serving.

Nutritional info: (per brownie)

- Calories: 200

- Fat: 9g

- Carbohydrates: 30g

- Fiber: 2g

- Protein: 2g

Peanut Butter Energy Balls

Description: Nutrient-packed energy balls
made with wholesome ingredients like oats,
peanut butter, and honey.

Preparation time: 10 minutes

Chilling time: 30 minutes

Number of servings: 12 balls

Ingredients:

- 1 cup rolled oats

- 1/2 cup creamy peanut butter

- 1/4 cup honey or maple syrup

- 1/4 cup mini chocolate chips

- 1/4 cup chopped nuts (such as almonds or walnuts)

- 1 teaspoon vanilla extract

- Pinch of salt

How to make:

1. In a large mixing bowl, combine the rolled oats, peanut butter, honey or maple syrup,

mini chocolate chips, chopped nuts, vanilla extract, and a pinch of salt.

2. Stir until all the ingredients are well combined and form a sticky dough.

3. Scoop tablespoonfuls of the dough and roll them into balls using your hands.

4. Place the energy balls on a baking sheet lined with parchment paper.

5. Chill the energy balls in the refrigerator for at least 30 minutes to firm up.

6. Once chilled, store the energy balls in an airtight container in the refrigerator for up to one week.

Nutritional info: (per ball)

- Calories: 120

- Fat: 7g

- Carbohydrates: 12g

- Fiber: 2g

- Protein: 4g

Lemon Cashew Cheesecake Bars

Description: Creamy and tangy cheesecake bars with a refreshing lemon flavor, made with a cashew-based filling and a gluten-free crust.

Preparation time: 20 minutes

Chilling time: 4 hours

Number of servings: 9 bars

Ingredients:

For the crust:

- 1 cup almond flour

- 1/4 cup coconut oil, melted

- 2 tablespoons maple syrup

- Pinch of salt

For the filling:

- 2 cups raw cashews, soaked in water for at least 4 hours or overnight

- 1/2 cup coconut cream

- 1/3 cup lemon juice

- 1/4 cup maple syrup

- 1/4 cup coconut oil, melted

- 1 teaspoon vanilla extract

- Zest of 1 lemon

How to make:

1. Line an 8x8-inch baking dish with parchment paper, leaving some overhang on the sides for easy removal.

2. In a medium bowl, combine the almond flour, melted coconut oil, maple syrup, and a pinch of salt. Mix until the ingredients are well combined and the mixture resembles coarse crumbs.

3. Press the crust mixture evenly into the bottom of the prepared baking dish. Place it in the freezer while you prepare the filling.

4. In a blender, combine the soaked cashews, coconut cream, lemon juice, maple syrup, melted coconut oil, vanilla extract, and lemon zest. Blend until smooth and creamy.

5. Pour the filling over the crust in the baking dish and spread it out evenly with a spatula.

6. Tap the dish gently on the counter to remove any air bubbles.

7. Place the cheesecake bars in the refrigerator and chill for at least 4 hours, or until set.

8. Once set, lift the cheesecake bars out of the baking dish using the parchment paper overhang. Slice into bars and serve chilled.

9. Store any leftovers in an airtight container in the refrigerator for up to one week.

Nutritional info: (per bar)

- Calories: 300

- Fat: 24g

- Carbohydrates: 18g

- Fiber: 2g

- Protein: 6g

Chocolate Avocado Truffles

Description: Rich and creamy chocolate truffles made with ripe avocados for a healthier twist on a classic treat.

Preparation time: 15 minutes

Chilling time: 1 hour

Number of servings: 12 truffles

Ingredients:

- 2 ripe avocados, peeled and pitted

- 1/4 cup cocoa powder

- 1/4 cup maple syrup or honey

- 1 teaspoon vanilla extract

- Pinch of salt

- Shredded coconut, cocoa powder, or chopped nuts for coating (optional)

How to make:

1. In a food processor, combine the ripe avocados, cocoa powder, maple syrup or honey, vanilla extract, and a pinch of salt.

2. Blend until smooth and creamy, scraping down the sides of the bowl as needed.

3. Transfer the chocolate avocado mixture to a bowl and refrigerate for 30 minutes to firm up.

4. Once chilled, scoop tablespoonfuls of the mixture and roll them into balls using your hands.

5. If desired, roll the truffles in shredded coconut, cocoa powder, or chopped nuts to coat.

6. Place the coated truffles on a baking sheet lined with parchment paper.

7. Chill the truffles in the refrigerator for at least 30 minutes before serving.

Nutritional info: (per truffle)

- Calories: 70

- Fat: 5g

- Carbohydrates: 7g

- Fiber: 2g

- Protein: 1g

Vegan Apple Crisp

Description: Warm and comforting apple crisp topped with a crispy oat topping, made without butter or dairy.

Preparation time: 15 minutes

Baking time: 40 minutes

Number of servings: 6

Ingredients:

For the filling:

- 4 large apples, peeled, cored, and sliced

- 2 tablespoons maple syrup

- 1 tablespoon lemon juice

- 1 teaspoon ground cinnamon

- 1/4 teaspoon ground nutmeg

For the topping:

- 1 cup rolled oats

- 1/2 cup almond flour

- 1/4 cup chopped nuts (such as walnuts or pecans)

- 1/4 cup coconut oil, melted

- 1/4 cup maple syrup

- 1 teaspoon ground cinnamon

- Pinch of salt

How to make:

1. Preheat your oven to 350°F (175°C). Grease an 8x8-inch baking dish.

2. In a large bowl, toss together the sliced apples, maple syrup, lemon juice, ground cinnamon, and ground nutmeg until the apples are evenly coated. Transfer the apple mixture to the prepared baking dish.

3. In the same bowl (no need to clean it), combine the rolled oats, almond flour, chopped nuts, melted coconut oil, maple syrup, ground cinnamon, and a pinch of salt. Mix until the ingredients are well combined and form a crumbly mixture.

4. Sprinkle the oat topping evenly over the apples in the baking dish.

5. Bake in the preheated oven for 35-40 minutes, or until the topping is golden brown and the apples are tender.

6. Remove from the oven and let it cool for a few minutes before serving.

7. Serve the vegan apple crisp warm, optionally with a scoop of dairy-free vanilla ice cream.

Nutritional info: (per serving)

- Calories: 280

- Fat: 12g

- Carbohydrates: 41g

- Fiber: 6g

- Protein: 4g

Mango Chia Pudding Parfaits

Description: Creamy mango chia pudding layered with fresh mango chunks and granola for a delicious and nutritious breakfast or snack.

Preparation time: 10 minutes

Chilling time: 4 hours (or overnight)

Number of servings: 2

Ingredients:

- 1 ripe mango, peeled, pitted, and diced

- 1 cup unsweetened almond milk (or any plant-based milk)

- 1/4 cup chia seeds

- 1 tablespoon maple syrup or honey (optional)

- Granola, for layering

- Fresh berries, for topping (optional)

- Shredded coconut, for garnish (optional)

How to make:

1. In a blender, combine half of the diced mango and the almond milk. Blend until smooth.

2. Transfer the mango mixture to a bowl and stir in the chia seeds and maple syrup or honey, if using. Mix well.

3. Cover the bowl and refrigerate the mango chia pudding for at least 4 hours, or preferably overnight, to allow it to thicken.

4. Once the chia pudding has set, assemble the parfaits by layering the pudding with the remaining diced mango and granola in serving glasses or jars.

5. Top the parfaits with fresh berries and shredded coconut, if desired.

6. Serve chilled and enjoy!

Nutritional info: (per serving)

- Calories: 250

- Fat: 9g

- Carbohydrates: 38g

- Fiber: 11g

- Protein: 6g

Strawberry Nice Cream

Description: Creamy and luscious "ice cream" made from frozen bananas and strawberries, with no added sugar.

Preparation time: 5 minutes

Freezing time: 4 hours (or until solid)

Number of servings: 4

Ingredients:

- 4 ripe bananas, peeled, sliced, and frozen

- 2 cups frozen strawberries

- 1 teaspoon vanilla extract

- Fresh strawberries, for garnish (optional)

- Mint leaves, for garnish (optional)

How to make:

1. In a food processor or high-speed blender, combine the frozen banana slices, frozen strawberries, and vanilla extract.

2. Blend until smooth and creamy, scraping down the sides of the bowl as needed.

3. If the nice cream is too thick, you can add a splash of plant-based milk to help it blend.

4. Once the mixture is smooth and creamy, transfer it to a freezer-safe container and freeze for at least 4 hours, or until solid.

5. When ready to serve, let the nice cream sit at room temperature for a few minutes to soften slightly.

6. Scoop the strawberry nice cream into bowls and garnish with fresh strawberries and mint leaves, if desired.

7. Serve immediately and enjoy!

Nutritional info: (per serving)

- Calories: 150

- Fat: 1g

- Carbohydrates: 38g

- Fiber: 6g

- Protein: 2g

Chocolate Banana Popsicles

Description: Creamy and indulgent chocolate popsicles made with bananas, cocoa powder, and coconut milk.

Preparation time: 10 minutes

Freezing time: 4 hours

Number of servings: 6 popsicles

Ingredients:

- 2 ripe bananas

- 1/4 cup cocoa powder

- 1 cup full-fat coconut milk

- 2 tablespoons maple syrup or honey

- 1 teaspoon vanilla extract

- Pinch of salt

- Popsicle molds

How to make:

1. In a blender, combine the ripe bananas, cocoa powder, coconut milk, maple syrup or honey, vanilla extract, and a pinch of salt.

2. Blend until smooth and creamy.

3. Pour the chocolate banana mixture into popsicle molds, leaving a little space at the top for expansion.

4. Insert popsicle sticks into the molds.

5. Place the popsicle molds in the freezer and freeze for at least 4 hours, or until the popsicles are solid.

6. Once frozen, remove the popsicles from the molds by running them under warm water for a few seconds.

7. Serve the chocolate banana popsicles immediately and enjoy!

Nutritional info: (per popsicle)

- Calories: 120

- Fat: 6g

- Carbohydrates: 17g

- Fiber: 3g

- Protein: 2g

Conclusion

As you've journeyed through the pages of this book, you've likely discovered a newfound appreciation for the incredible diversity and flavors that the plant kingdom has to offer. From vibrant veggies and luscious fruits to hearty grains, legumes, and meat alternatives, the possibilities for creating delicious and nutritious plant-based meals are truly endless.

Perhaps you've surprised yourself by falling in love with dishes you never imagined you'd enjoy, like a rich and creamy dairy-free pasta sauce or a decadent vegan brownie that's every bit as indulgent as its traditional counterpart. Or maybe you've rediscovered the simple joys of roasting vegetables to bring out their natural sweetness or tossing together a fresh, colorful salad that's as beautiful as it is nourishing.

Regardless of where your plant-based journey began, one thing is certain: you now possess the knowledge and skills to continue exploring this way of eating with confidence and creativity. The recipes and meal plans in this book have provided a solid foundation, but they're merely the beginning. Feel empowered to experiment, to swap out ingredients based on your personal preferences or what's in season, and to constantly seek out new flavors and combinations that excite your palate.

Remember, a plant-based lifestyle isn't about deprivation or restriction – it's about embracing the abundance and diversity that nature has to offer. It's about nourishing your body with whole, nutrient-dense foods that provide sustained energy, support optimal health, and promote a sense of overall well-being.

As you continue on this path, you may find that the benefits extend far beyond your own physical health. By making more conscious, planet-friendly food choices, you're playing a vital role in protecting the environment and preserving natural resources for generations to come. Your simple act of embracing a plant-based diet is a powerful act of compassion and sustainability.

So, keep exploring, keep experimenting, and keep savoring the incredible flavors and textures that plant-based cuisine has to offer. This book has merely scratched the surface – the rest is up to you and your own culinary journey. Here's to a lifetime of vibrant, nourishing, and delicious plant-based meals!

www.ingramcontent.com/pod-product-compliance
Lightning Source LLC
Chambersburg PA
CBHW061620250726
48659CB00004B/1022